ACSM Health Fitness Specialist Study Guide

Test Prep Secrets for the ACSM CHFS

Printed in the United States of America

Table of Contents

Introduction

Congratulations on your decision to pursue an American College of Sports Medicine Health Fitness Specialist certification!

Whether this is your first certification or your fifth, no one makes the choice to become certified without first researching the certifying agency. Numerous certifications exist, but few are widely recognized. ACSM certifications are internationally recognized and are considered by many to be the "gold standard" by which other certifications are judged.

But, is ACSM certification the best for you and your future goals? How difficult is the test? Does it really matter what certification you have? Can you learn the material and apply it when it really counts?

Don't let doubts and fear stand in the way of pursuing your dreams! This book will answer all of your questions, and help you put those doubts to bed once and for all. Within these pages you can expect to find, not only answers to these common questions, but also crucial details that will help you achieve the ACSM HFS certification.

We will review material that you can expect to see at test time, and offer tips and tricks that will help you feel confident in your ability to apply what you know in practice.

Why Should I Get Certified through the ACSM?
Good question! When gaining your certification, you want to make sure that you are going to receive the maximum benefit for your choice.

To start off, let's first take a look at the American College of Sports Medicine. The ACSM is the largest sports medicine and exercise science organization in the world, with over 45,000 members and certified professionals. As an internationally recognized body, the ACSM is widely respected as an agency that promotes research in the field of exercise science and applies that research in practical applications.

Where Can I Find Work?
Certified Health Fitness Specialists work with both physically healthy individuals, as well as those who suffer from chronic conditions that are currently being controlled. Performing pre-exercise screenings and interpreting results of these assessments is an integral part of the CFHS duties.

As a fitness and health specialist, you will create exercise prescriptions for individuals based on their unique circumstances. You will use behavior and motivational techniques to help clients learn to change behaviors in an effort to improve their health and wellness.

According the US Bureau of Labor Statistics, fitness and exercise specialists can look forward to more job opportunities if they obtain certification in their chosen specialty. Certified Health Fitness Specialists often find employment at universities, hospitals, and in other corporate environments. Some specialists choose to work independently and find private clients.

All American College of Sports Medicine certifications are administered by Pearson VUE at one of 5,000 testing locations worldwide. The certification exam is computer based and is scored on a pass or fail basis.

So, ready to get started?

Important Information: Registering for the Exam

The American College of Sports Medicine requires that candidates for certification undergo examination at a Pearson VUE testing center. Pearson VUE testing is computer-based, and the tests are given on demand. Candidates for certification should register with Pearson VUE at least **24 hours** prior to testing.

Eligibility Requirements
In order to sit for the ACSM Health Fitness Specialist certification examination, candidates must:

- Possess a Bachelor's degree, or be in the last semester to complete a Bachelor's degree or higher, in kinesiology, exercise physiology, exercise science, or a related major.

- Be currently certified in adult CPR/AED with a practical component.

Fees
As with all certifications, fees will be assessed prior to testing.

- ACSM members pay $219.00.
- Non-ACSM members pay $279.00.
- Fee for re-testing is $150.00.

Non-ACSM members can join the American College of Sports Medicine prior to registering for the exam and receive a voucher to pay the discounted fee. To become a member of the ACSM, visit their website at www.acsm.org.

Registration for the Exam
Eligible candidates can register for the ACSM certification examination in one of three ways:

- By telephone: Call Pearson VUE at 888-VUE-ACSM, Monday through Friday from 7:00 AM to 7:00 PM.
- In person: If you are local to a Pearson VUE testing center you may choose to register in person.
- Online: Visit the ACSM certification site (http://certification.acsm.org) and navigate to the correct area of the Pearson VUE site.

Important Note: Regardless of registration method, candidates are strongly encouraged to register at least **24 hours** prior to their testing time in order to ensure correct username and password verification. Candidates failing to register at least 24 hours prior to test administration may not be allowed to test at their chosen time due to space availability.

Test Duration and Scoring
You will be allowed 3½ hours to complete the examination. The test consists of 150 test questions. Twenty-five of the questions on the test will not be scored; these are test questions that are being considered for future test purposes. Because it is impossible to know which questions asked are test questions, treat every question as though it will be scored.

ACSM pre-determines passing scores for all certification examinations. A passing score is 550 on a scale of 200 to 800.

Results

You will receive your test results immediately upon completing the certification examination. Those who have successfully completed the exam will receive their certification in the mail in approximately six to eight weeks. Also included will be an ACSM certification wallet card.

Unsuccessful candidates will also be notified of their failing grade immediately upon completion, and a voucher to re-test will be provided by Pearson VUE to candidates who wish to test again. Re-tests can be scheduled every 15 days from the prior exam date until successful certification.

Breaking Down the ACSM Health Fitness Specialist Exam

The ACSM Health Fitness Specialist certification examination is divided into 10 domains. The domain and the approximate percentages of test questions relating to each domain are listed below.

1. Health Appraisal and Fitness Exercise Testing (12%). 18
2. Exercise Prescription and Programming (31%). 46 -
3. Exercise Physiology and Related Exercise Science (23%). 34 -
4. Nutrition and Weight Management (8%). 12
5. Program Administration and Outcomes Assessment (8%). 12
6. Safety, Injury Prevention, and Emergency Procedures (7%). 10
7. Human Behavior (4%). 6
8. Electrocardiography and Diagnostic Techniques (1%). 2 -
9. Medical and Surgical Management (1%). 2 -
10. Pathophysiology and Risk Factors (5%). 8 -

Candidates who sit for the exam should be thoroughly knowledgeable about all domains listed, and have a solid grasp of the fundamentals regarding human anatomy and exercise movements. For ACSM Health Fitness Specialist certification, it isn't enough to simply memorize material. You must be able to apply the knowledge in various situations.

How Is the Test Scored?

As previously mentioned, only 125 of the 150 questions on the exam will be used to calculate your final score. The test is graded on a pass or fail basis, and the passing score is set in advance for all ACSM certification exams. You **must** receive a score of 550 or higher to become certified. Tests are graded on a scale ranging from 200 – 800 points.

Chapter 1: Let's Make a Plan

Just as you wouldn't advise a client to jump right into a rigorous exercise program without first warming up, it makes little sense to dive head-first into test material without preparing to make the most of what you study.

Create a Study Plan

Organize Your Tools: Keep your study material in a set location. Having notes sprawled across the house isn't helpful, and you're likely to lose important information at some point. Whether it is a designated drawer, box, or corner of a desk, find a place to store all of your material together.

Write Down Information: Regardless of whether you feel you learn best by hearing information or seeing information, write it down. The act of writing down important notes will require you to focus on each fact and help you remember the information when it's needed most – test day!

Break-Out the Highlighters: Don't settle for just one color. Use a variety of colored highlighters to help you piece together information as you study. For example, use a pink highlighter for information you need to remember regarding the circulatory system, and use blue to accentuate information regarding injury prevention. Create a color system and stick to it.

Use the Calendar: Just as you will be asking your clients to schedule appropriate times for exercise, you must schedule time to study. Remember, you wouldn't ask your client to do things you wouldn't or couldn't do, right? Dedicate time for study every week.

Take Time for Play: All work and no play makes Jack a dull boy, and all study with no break makes you stressed out, irritable, and probably not too fun to be around! Scheduling breaks, or even days, off from studying will allow you to let the material you've been poring over sink in a bit, and you will retain more information when you approach it in a relaxed state.

Nourish Your Brain: This isn't the time to go on a crash diet, or start restricting calories! Be sure to eat well and keep a nice supply of brain-boosting super foods on hand to snack on. You won't concentrate well if your tummy is rumbling, so remember to eat right and avoid caffeine overloads in hopes of staying alert as you prepare.

Sleep Is Important: Avoid late-night study sessions that will leave you all blurry-eyed in the morning. Many people find that their brain tends to turn over difficult problems through the night while sleeping, and when they awake the next day, they understand the issue more clearly. Even if this doesn't work for you, being exhausted won't help your mental clarity.

Draw It Out: If you learn best by seeing flow-charts or diagrams, by all means, grab some paper and sketch out the details. Add color for emphasis if you need to - just don't let yourself get caught up in your artwork as opposed to your true purpose of learning the material you color!

Keep It Quiet: Be certain that you study in as quiet a location as possible. Turn off the television, radio, and cell phones. Eliminate as many distractions as you can. You can always check for messages or listen to a few tunes during a study break, but don't let these things eat up your scheduled study times.

Note What You Don't Understand: In the event that you run across information that you simply cannot grasp, make a note of this and continue your studies. Don't stop just because you don't understand one point. You will likely find that a piece of information presented later will bring the bigger picture into focus. The worst case scenario here would be that you are left with a few items that you need to research for true clarification.

Enlist the Help of Friends and Family: Though very few questions on the certification exam will call for total recall of a fact or definition, let friends and family help you in your quest for certification. Make some flashcards that list various medical issues you will likely encounter in your clients, and another set that deals with exercise physiology. Have study helpers to choose a card from each pile and explain how you would handle the client with these issues. If you don't know or aren't sure about a given scenario, make a note of that and study that point during your next study session.

What to Do on Test Day

Get Up Early: Plan to get up early on test day if you registered for a morning certification exam. Give yourself plenty of time to shower and dress appropriately for the day. You need not feel compelled to wear your Sunday best, but remember that confidence is crucial on test day, and you will feel more confident wearing clean, comfortable clothes.

Don't Skip Breakfast: Get your day off to the right start, even if you aren't testing until later in the afternoon. Keeping your body fueled properly will ensure that your brain is functioning well when test time arrives.

Have a Small Snack Before the Test: Remember, this test lasts for 3½ hours. You won't concentrate well if you're looking forward to the next meal because you're already hungry. Eat light, and don't go overboard with the liquids, either. It's nearly impossible to concentrate when your bladder is filled to capacity!

Know Where You're Going: If you aren't positive of the testing location, be sure to print out directions which include alternate routes around high traffic areas. You must arrive on time for your appointment else you risk not being admitted. Leave home early enough to allow for traffic delays and congestion.

Arrive to the Testing Center Early: No one likes feeling rushed, and you probably won't fare well if you sit down for a comprehensive examination that can determine your future feeling flustered. Plan to arrive at the testing location between 15 to 30 minutes prior to your appointment time.

What to Bring: You will be **required** to show identification before being allowed to test. You will need two forms of ID: Primary and Secondary.

1. <u>Primary Identification</u>
    - Your primary identification must have a fixed photo. A driver's license, school or employee identification badge, and some credit cards which have your photo attached will work as a primary ID. The identification must be valid and not expired.

2. <u>Secondary Identification</u>
    - Secondary identification must contain a valid signature. Consider bringing a signed credit card, Social Security card, or passport. Again, the identification must be valid and not expired.

Consider Bringing: A number of items considered "comfort items" may be allowed in the testing center by test administrators. Examples of comfort items include:

- Cough drops and tissues.
- Sweaters or sweatshirts.
- Eye glasses or hearing aids.
- Pillows for back support, or to support an injured limb.
- Neck braces for those with neck injuries.

Important Note: Be certain to ask test administrators for permission to bring comfort items into the testing center. Do not assume these items will be allowed.

Do NOT Bring:

- Purses, wallets, briefcases, or backpacks.
- Coats or jackets.
- Study materials.
- Electronic devices, including pagers and cell phones.
- Food or drinks.

Calculators will be provided on the testing computer as needed. Certification candidates will not be allowed to use note paper or any pens or pencils that are not provided by the test administrator. A small white board and erasable marker will be provided by the testing facility should you need to make any notations during your exam.

After the Exam

You will learn of the results of your certification examination immediately after submitting your test. Candidates who successfully completed the test will receive a welcome packet from the American College of Sports Medicine in approximately six to eight weeks after the exam results are received by the organization. Within the packet will be your certification and a wallet card.

Upon passing certification testing, the ACSM allows you to make your contact information publicly available on their website via the Pro-Finder. If you had successfully completed certification previously, you can still utilize the Pro-Finder by "opting in" on the ACSM website.

Candidates who were unsuccessful in passing will be given a voucher for re-testing by the test administrator at the Pearson VUE testing site. You may re-take the certification test following a 15 day period from the exam date. The cost for re-testing is $150.00.

Chapter 2: Health Appraisal and Fitness Exercise Testing

Before you can begin prescribing treatments and exercise programs, you must first ascertain the needs of your patient. Having the proper knowledge, skills, and abilities for Health Appraisal and Fitness Exercise Testing is absolutely essential.

HEALTH APPRAISAL

Pretest Considerations for Health Appraisal

Health fitness professionals must be both well-trained and knowledgeable in client-health risk appraisal, a systematic approach in screening clients for: signs and symptoms, a family history of, and risk factors for disease. New clients, especially, will need to fill out and use a variety of forms. Information drawn from the screening can help identify:

- Contraindications to exercise. In the presence of contraindications, the health fitness professional should determine whether or not the client may still participate in an exercise program.

- Individuals who must undergo additional exercise testing – and even a medical evaluation – because of an increased risk for disease due to age, symptoms, and/or additional risk factors.

- Those who should participate only in medically-supervised exercise programs, due to the presence of a clinically significant disease.

- Any other person who may have special considerations.

In the presence of any of the above, clients would require a medical evaluation before engaging in a fitness program. They may even need medical supervision while exercising.

Informed Consent

Before any exercise testing or health appraisals can begin, patients must provide a form which indicates their own informed consent. (An example can be found on the following page.) This form stresses the risks and benefits of exercise testing and programming, while stating those occurrences which are possible during testing, such as risks, side effects, etc.

Clients must always be fully aware of testing or exercise procedures and their risks; the signed informed consent form serves as both a legal and ethical document in these regards.

INFORMED CONSENT

I hereby consent to participate in the outpatient exercise at ________________________.

I understand that I will be placed on a program of graded exercise and activities. The levels of exercise I will do will be based on my cardiovascular response. Regularly scheduled sessions will be held for the purpose of evaluating my progress. Explicit instructions regarding the amount and kind of exercises and activities I should do will be provided. My daily exercise program will be based on my pulse rate response and level of exertion during the treatment sessions.

I understand that there exists a possibility of certain changes during the exercise session. These changes include abnormal blood pressure, heart dysrhythmias, fainting, and in very rare circumstances heart attack or even death. I understand that every effort will be made to minimize these problems by obtaining a thorough medical history and observations during the exercise sessions.

I realize it is necessary for me to promptly report to the exercise physiologist any signs or symptoms indicating discomfort or distress. I consent to the administration of any immediate resuscitation measures deemed advisable by the supervisor of the exercise session and/or any other qualified medical personnel present at the time.

No assurance has been given to me that this rehabilitation program will increase my functional activity level. The results may help in evaluating what types of activity I may carry out safely in my daily life.

I have read and understand the above information. Any questions which have arisen have been answered to my satisfaction.

Participant signature_______________________________ Date________________________

Witness signature__________________________________ Date________________________

PAR-Q

An effective, safe, and commonly-used form for screening is the **Physical Activity Readiness Questionnaire (PAR-Q)** form. The PAR- Q has been recommended as a minimal standard for entry into moderate-intensity exercise programs; it was designed to identify the small number of adults for whom physical activity might be inappropriate or who should receive medical advice concerning the most suitable type of activity.

The PAR-Q requires clients to fill out a seven-question questionnaire regarding their health. If a client answers "yes" to any of the questions on the form, then you are required to obtain a consent form (also known as a **Medical Release** form) from that client's healthcare provider before beginning an exercise program. All clients must also sign the **Informed Consent** and **Release of Liability** forms, which are often combined into a single form.

You may or may not, depending on the client, require the completion of other forms to add specificity and coherency to a client's profile. These can include: Orthopedic History, Nutritional Profile, Past and Current Activity History, Exercise Attitude Questionnaire, etc.

The information gathered in the screening is used by health fitness professionals for a variety of purposes: making recommendations for lifestyle modifications, suggesting strategies for exercise testing, prescribing exercise prescriptions, etc.

Physician Referral

As you will see, The PAR-Q states that clients should obtain medical clearance from their physician prior to starting an exercise program. This is a safeguard for high-risk clients who may compromise their health by exercising in a facility without medically-trained staff and necessary equipment.

Some patients may indicate a risk or contraindication to testing. In those cases, you need to refer your patient to their physician for further testing specifically regarding those contraindications. This is mandatory for further clinical testing, as well as for when the client requires medical clearance into an office- or hospital-based program (or medical fitness center).

The physician can provide a formal referral form, or simply a doctor's office script with the physician's name, stating the diagnosis and exercise prescription.

Physical Activity Readiness Questionnaire - PAR-Q (revised 2002)

PAR-Q & YOU

(A Questionnaire for People Aged 15 to 69)

Regular physical activity is fun and healthy, and increasingly more people are starting to become more active every day. Being more active is very safe for most people. However, some people should check with their doctor before they start becoming much more physically active.

If you are planning to become much more physically active than you are now, start by answering the seven questions in the box below. If you are between the ages of 15 and 69, the PAR-Q will tell you if you should check with your doctor before you start. If you are over 69 years of age, and you are not used to being very active, check with your doctor.

Common sense is your best guide when you answer these questions. Please read the questions carefully and answer each one honestly: check YES or NO.

YES	NO	
☐	☐	**1. Has your doctor ever said that you have a heart condition and that you should only do physical activity recommended by a doctor?**
☐	☐	**2. Do you feel pain in your chest when you do physical activity?**
☐	☐	**3. In the past month, have you had chest pain when you were not doing physical activity?**
☐	☐	**4. Do you lose your balance because of dizziness or do you ever lose consciousness?**
☐	☐	**5. Do you have a bone or joint problem (for example, back, knee or hip) that could be made worse by a change in your physical activity?**
☐	☐	**6. Is your doctor currently prescribing drugs (for example, water pills) for your blood pressure or heart condition?**
☐	☐	**7. Do you know of any other reason why you should not do physical activity?**

If you answered

YES to one or more questions

Talk with your doctor by phone or in person BEFORE you start becoming much more physically active or BEFORE you have a fitness appraisal. Tell your doctor about the PAR-Q and which questions you answered YES.

- You may be able to do any activity you want — as long as you start slowly and build up gradually. Or, you may need to restrict your activities to those which are safe for you. Talk with your doctor about the kinds of activities you wish to participate in and follow his/her advice.
- Find out which community programs are safe and helpful for you.

NO to all questions

If you answered NO honestly to all PAR-Q questions, you can be reasonably sure that you can:

- start becoming much more physically active – begin slowly and build up gradually. This is the safest and easiest way to go.
- take part in a fitness appraisal – this is an excellent way to determine your basic fitness so that you can plan the best way for you to live actively. It is also highly recommended that you have your blood pressure evaluated. If your reading is over 144/94, talk with your doctor before you start becoming much more physically active.

DELAY BECOMING MUCH MORE ACTIVE:

- if you are not feeling well because of a temporary illness such as a cold or a fever – wait until you feel better; or
- if you are or may be pregnant – talk to your doctor before you start becoming more active.

PLEASE NOTE: If your health changes so that you then answer YES to any of the above questions, tell your fitness or health professional. Ask whether you should change your physical activity plan.

Informed Use of the PAR-Q: The Canadian Society for Exercise Physiology, Health Canada, and their agents assume no liability for persons who undertake physical activity, and if in doubt after completing this questionnaire, consult your doctor prior to physical activity.

No changes permitted. You are encouraged to photocopy the PAR-Q but only if you use the entire form.

NOTE: If the PAR-Q is being given to a person before he or she participates in a physical activity program or a fitness appraisal, this section may be used for legal or administrative purposes.

"I have read, understood and completed this questionnaire. Any questions I had were answered to my full satisfaction."

NAME ____

SIGNATURE ____ DATE ____________________

SIGNATURE OF PARENT or GUARDIAN (for participants under the age of majority) ____________________ WITNESS ____________________

Note: This physical activity clearance is valid for a maximum of 12 months from the date it is completed and becomes invalid if your condition changes so that you would answer YES to any of the seven questions.

ACSM Risk Stratification

The PAR-Q is a quick form which, though effective, covers general information. A more comprehensive process of determining a patient's risk is through the ACSM Risk Stratification method. **Risk stratification** assigns individuals to low, medium, or high risk, based on presence of conditions. We will go over how to recognize the conditions, signs, and symptoms of various disease states later in this chapter.

The American College of Sports Medicine has a comprehensive approach in identifying any risk factors that your client might have: the **ACSM Risk Stratification Matrix**, which makes recommendations based upon the category (Low, Moderate, or High Risk) into which your client falls.

ACSM Risk Stratification is determined by adding up the number of risk factors indicated by clients during their screenings.

Positive Risk Factors

- **Family History of Disease**: Myocardial infarction, coronary revascularization, or sudden death before the age of 55 (for male first-degree relatives) or 65 (female first-degree relatives) years of age.

- **Cigarette Smoking**: Includes those with a current smoking habit, as well as those who have recently (within six months) quit and those who have been exposed to second-hand smoke for over six months.

- **Hypertension**: Those currently taking antihypertensive medication, and/or those who have a confirmed (by at least two separate measurements on two separate occasions) systolic blood pressure ≥ 140 mm Hg or diastolic ≥ 90 mm Hg.

- **Hypercholesterolemia/Dyslipidemia**: Those currently taking lipid-lowering medication, and/or those with a total serum cholesterol > 200 mg/dL (5.2 mmol/L), or high-density lipoprotein cholesterol of .35 mg/dL (0.9 mmol/L).[1]

- **Impaired Fasting Glucose**: A fasting blood glucose≥ 110 mg/dL (6.1 mmol/L, confirmed by at least two separate measurements on two separate occasions).

- **Obesity**: BMI ≥ 30 mg/m^2, or a waist girth exceeding approximately 39.4 inches.

- **Sedentary Lifestyle**: Those not meeting the recommended amount of physical activity as provided by the U.S. Surgeon General's Report. Typical Recommendation: At least 30 minutes of physical activity at a moderate intensity (40 – 60% VO2), at least three days a weeks, for at least three months

Negative Risk Factors

- **High Serum HDL Cholesterol**: > 60 mg/dL (1.6 mmol/L).

Emerging Risk Factors

- **Inflammatory Markers**: i.e., Reactive C Protein (CRP) and fibrinogen.

[1] Low-density lipoprotein cholesterol measurement is preferred over total cholesterol.

Once you've ascertained the amount of indications to any of the above given by your client, you may then classify them into one of the three categories, which also depend on the client's age:

Low Risk
Men < 45 years of age and women < 55 years of age, who are asymptomatic while meeting no more than one risk factor.

Moderate Risk
Men > 45 years and women > 55 years, or those who meet the threshold for two or more risk factors.

High Risk
Individuals with one or more signs and symptoms listed or a known cardiovascular, pulmonary, or metabolic disease.

These categories also come in handy for determining an appropriate level of exercise testing.

The following chart was taken from ronjones.org "High-Performance Health" (available in the public domain):

ACSM Recommendations for (A) Current Medical Examination[2] & Exercise Testing Prior to Participation and (B) Physician Supervision of Exercise Tests

	Low Risk	Moderate Risk	High Risk
A.			
Moderate Exercise	Not Necessary	Not Necessary	Recommended
Vigorous Exercise	Not Necessary	Recommended	Recommended
B.			
Submaximal Test	Not Necessary	Not Necessary	Recommended
Maximal Test	Not Necessary	Recommended	Recommended

Alternatively, you can classify your patient according to these categories:

Low Risk: Assumed when each of the below is present.

- No significant LVD (EF > 50%).
- No resting or exercised-induced complex dysrhythmias.
- No complications with any of the following: MI, CABG, PTCA, atherectomy, and/or stent.
    - Absence of CHF or signs/symptoms indicating post-event ischemia.
- Normal hemodynamics with exercise and recovery.
- Patient is asymptomatic, which includes the absence of angina with exertion or recovery.
- Function capacity ≥ METS (if n/a, don't use FWC to determine risk).
- Absence of clinical depression.

[2] Within the Past Year

Moderate Risk: Assumed for patients classified as neither highest nor lowest risk.

- Moderately-impaired LV function (EF = 40 – 50%).
- Angina signs and symptoms during moderate levels of exercise (5 – 6.9 METs) or during recovery.
- Those with abnormal resting EKGs, including: LBBB; LVH, with or without resting ST-T changes; non-specific intraventricular conduction delays; WPW; and ventricular paced rhythms.
- Those on digitalis therapy.
- Those with tests negative for ischemia who fail to achieve 85% of maximal predicted heart rate.

High Risk: Assumed with the presence of any one of the risk factors included in this category.

- Decreased LV function (EF < 40%).
- Survivor of cardiac arrest or sudden death.
- Complex ventricular dysrhythmia, at rest or with exercise.
- MI or cardiac surgery complicated by cardiogenic shock, CHF, and/or signs and symptoms of post-procedure ischemia.
- Abnormal hemodynamics with exercise (especially flat or decreasing SBP or chronotropic incompetence with increasing workload).
- Signs and symptoms indicating angina pectoris at low levels of exercise (< 5.0 METs) or in recovery.
- Function capacity < 5.0 METs (if FWC n/a, don't use this variable to consider risk).
- Clinically-significant depression.

FITNESS EXERCISE TESTING

While almost anyone can exercise safely, some people may benefit from an exercise consultation. The top two reasons to get exercise prescriptions are safety and efficiency. An exercise program needs to be designed specifically for health status, goals, abilities, and interests. When working with clients who are healthy, you will generally only need informed consent before developing exercise prescriptions for them; each exercise program will need to suit the client's current fitness level.

When performing exercise testing for a patient, ACSM has certain steps, which can be put into the acronym "M.R.I.P.L."

"M" – Medical History
Ascertain the client's medical history through a series of questionnaires helps determine the following: the client's needs, special or otherwise; the necessity for a more extensive medical evaluation; and/or if the client ought to be referred to a different facility.

If clients end up staying at your facility, then you must also determine whether or not they have a clinical history which warrants modifying the typical prescription/program.

"R" – Risk Factor Assessment
The client needs to fill out a risk factor assessment form, identifying any health risk factors which would require a physician's approval before beginning a program. We will cover risk factors in greater depth later on, as well.

"I" – Interpreting the Data

At this stage, you should begin thinking about how best to design the client's exercise program. Once the client has completed their medical history and risk factor assessment forms, you must then assess the quality and completeness of the **fitness assessment**. At the clearance of their physician, the client will need to perform a fitness assessment, which should cover all **five components of fitness**:

1. Cardiovascular endurance.
2. Muscular strength.
3. Muscular endurance.
4. Flexibility.
5. Body composition.

We'll go into more detail regarding the fitness assessment later on the chapter.

Interpreting the data from this and the previous steps will help determine the client's health status, as well as identify specific goals and hurdles which ought to be considered in their exercise prescription.

"P" – Prescribing an Exercise Program

Now, you can develop your client's complete exercise prescription, appropriate for his or her current fitness level, which achieves a balance between goals and needs.

"L" – Lifestyle Counseling

This is perhaps one of the most important steps, which changes the exercise prescription from a temporary fix to the ideal: a lifestyle change. The client must be informed of the rationale underlying the developed program. It's helpful to review with them all the data from the previous M.R.I.P. steps, *specifically* and *in detail*; then, describe how your client can make the desired lifestyle changes, which includes an integration of the suggested exercise, dietary, and CVD risk factor reduction changes. Your instructions will need to be very thorough and clear and, depending on the client, must include directions for:

1. Modifying cardiovascular disease risk factors, including exercise and dietary changes.

2. Beginning an exercise program to reach goals.
   - For CV exercises, include modifications appropriate for the client's exercise and clinical history.
   - For weight loss, include an exercise program with dietary changes (with consideration to the Food Guide Pyramid, the Therapeutic Lifestyle Change Diet, and/or USDA Dietary Guidelines). U.S. Dept. of Agriculture
   - For a program of resistive exercise, include a consideration of the client's exercise and clinical history.

3. Referring your client to a specialist, when necessary, such as: a registered dietitian for dietary changes; a physician for prescribing lipid-lowering medications; or a counselor to assist with smoking cessation, stress management, etc.

Fitness Assessment: Risk Factors and Contraindications

In order to identify any underlying health issues which would limit a client's ability to exercise, a well-trained health fitness professional will usually require the client to undergo a general physical exam by their physician. Once the physician gives clearance, an appropriate exercise program can start being developed.

However, you may go beyond this and have your client participate in a fitness assessment (exercise testing) to establish the baseline of their current fitness level. This helps determine what types of exercise the client can perform safely.

An assessment often includes simple measurements of blood pressure and heart rate, as well as strength, flexibility (sit and reach test), body mass index (BMI), girth measurements, body fat percentage, cardiovascular endurance (3-minute step test), exercise history, and concludes with the client's own goals and interests. A graded exercise test, or **stress test**, will usually only be recommended by a physician if the client has symptoms of coronary artery diseases, or significant risk factors for CAD.

A screening tool, such as a **Par-Q** or **Health Status Questionnaire** (HSQ), may be used to quickly and accurately identify the following: medical contraindications to exercise, risk factors for coronary heart disease, and lifestyle behaviors which may affect your client's ability to exercise safely.

Risk Factors

Evidence supports an inverse relationship between physical activity and many disease states: cardiovascular disease (CVD); hypertension (HTN); stroke; osteoporosis; Type II diabetes mellitus (T2DM); obesity; colon cancer; breast cancer; anxiety; depression; etc.

Exercise does not provoke cardiovascular events in healthy individuals with normal cardiovascular systems. However, in certain individuals, vigorous exercise may result in cardiac arrest, or even sudden death. These individuals would have diagnosed or present cardiovascular diseases, congenital abnormalities, and/or hereditary abnormalities, such as:

- Hypertrophic cardiomyopathy.
- Coronary artery abnormalities (such as vessels that are abnormally narrow).
- Aortic stenosis.

Because of the prevalence of cardiac events in those populations, it is absolutely essential to screen for the presence of signs, symptoms, and risk factors of heart disease and other conditions.

The three most looked-for diseases – cardiovascular, pulmonary, and metabolic – include the following:

/peripheral artery disease

Cardiovascular Diseases: All cardiac, peripheral (PAD), vascular, and/or cerebrovascular diseases.

Pulmonary Diseases: Chronic obstructive pulmonary disease (COPD), asthma, interstitial lining disease, and/or cystic fibrosis.

Metabolic Diseases: Diabetes mellitus (Type I or II), thyroid disorders, renal disease, and/or liver disease. Symptoms can include: high blood sugar levels (sign of Diabetes Mellitus and obesity);

shakiness and disorientation (symptoms of hypoglycemia); weight gain, sluggish behavior, and hair loss (indicative of hypothyroidism)

The signs and symptoms of cardiovascular and pulmonary diseases include:

- Pain, discomfort, distress, or the equivalent, in areas which may be due to ischemia. Such areas include: chest, neck, jaw, arms, etc.

- Shortness of breath occurring at rest or with mild exertion.

- Dizziness or syncope. - fainting
- Known heart murmur
- Edema, especially of the ankle.

- Tachycardia, or other arrhythmic occurrences such as a known heart murmur. (heart beats >100 bpm)

- Orthopnea or paroxysmal dyspnea. (SOB when lying flat) SOB that occurs at night - "cardiac asthma"

- Intermittent claudication. muscle pain during exer (usually in calf)

- Unusual fatigue or shortness of breath with usual activities of daily life.

Aside from the big three, you must be familiar with the following conditions and their typical symptoms:

Angina
Heart Pain.

Symptoms Include: (Severity, type, and duration can vary.) Chest pain or discomfort; pain in arms, neck, jaw, shoulder, or back (accompanying chest pain); nausea; fatigue; shortness of breath; anxiety; sweating; and dizziness.

- **Stable Angina**: Most common type, occurring with exertion and going away with rest, though it can be triggered by mental or emotional stress. Could feel like indigestion, and may spread to arms, back, or other areas.

- **Unstable Angina**: A medical emergency, unstable angina occurs even at rest and is usually more severe and long-lasting than stable angina, sometimes lasting as long as 30 minutes. May signal a heart attack.

Arrhythmias
Abnormal heart rhythm.

- **Tachycardia**: Very fast heart rate. HR $\geq$ 100 bpm

- **Bradycardia**: Unusually slow heart rate. HR $<$ 60 bpm

- **Atrial Fibrillation**: Irregular heart rhythm.

- **Ventricular Ectopic Beats (VEB)**: A heart beat arising from an abnormal focus. Are called premature (occurring before the scheduled next beat) or escape (occurring later than the scheduled next beat) beats.

Dyspnea
Shortness of Breath (SOB). Difficult or uncomfortable breathing experienced subjectively (perceived and reported by patient). Can occur at rest, or be caused by exertion.

Exertion-caused Dyspnea suggests presence of cardiopulmonary disorders (especially left ventricular dysfunction or chronic obstructive pulmonary disease). Dyspnea should be differentiated from the following, which are indicative of respiratory variations that are not subjective:

- **Tachypnea**: Increase in respiratory rate above normal.
- **Hyperventilation**: Increased minute ventilation relative to metabolic need.
- **Hyperpnea**: Disproportionate rise in minute ventilation relative to an increase in metabolic level.

Important Note: Dyspnea on Exertion (DOE) may occur normally.

Edema
Swelling caused by excess fluid trapped in the body's tissues. Commonly occurs in the arms, hands, legs, ankles, and feet. Medication can be taken to remove excess fluid, and removing salt from the patient's diet typically relieves the swelling. However, edema can be a sign of an underlying disease (heart failure, kidney disease, cirrhosis of the liver, etc.).

Symptoms Include: Swelling or puffiness of the tissue directly under the skin, increased abdominal size, skin which appears stretched and/or shiny, and/or skin which retains a dimple after being pressed for several seconds.

formation of a blood clot inside a blood vessel

- **Unilateral Edema**: A limb which is completely swollen. Often results from venous thrombosis or lymphatic blockage in the limb.
- **Ankle Edema**: Most commonly-seen. A characteristic sign of heart failure or bilateral chronic venous insufficiency.

Heart Murmur
Usually harmless; however, heart murmurs can be caused by blood flowing through a damaged or overworked heart valve. This could indicate valvular abnormalities.

Intermittent Claudication
Refers to a muscle with inadequate blood supply being stressed by exercise, causing pain. Intermittent claudication does not occur when standing or sitting, and is reproducible from day to day; it is more severe when walking upstairs or up a hill.

Symptoms Include: Often described as a cramp. Disappears within one to two minutes after stopping exercise.

lying down

Orthopnea: A sensation of breathlessness that occurs in the recumbent position. Sensation is relieved by sitting or standing. Usually indicative of LV dysfunction.

Paroxysmal Nocturnal Dyspnea (PND)
Dyspnea which occurs usually after 1 or 2 hours of sleep.

Symptoms Include: Wheezing and coughing, which waken the sleeper. Can occur in COPDs. Oftentimes, the sleeper is relieved once awakening to either sit up or productively cough.

Syncope
Loss of consciousness, usually caused by reduced perfusion to the brain. When accompanied by vertigo– dizziness, syncope may result from cardiac disorders preventing normal cardiac output. These disorders include severe CAD, hypertrophic cardiomyopathy, aortic stenosis, and malignant ventricular dysrhythmias. Dizziness may also occur from loss of venous return to the heart.

Palpitations
Feelings of fluttering, rapid, or pounding heartbeats. Usually harmless, these can be triggered by: stress, exercise, or medication. However, palpitations may signify a greater cardiac disorder.

Symptoms Include: Perceived feelings of skipped, fluttering, too fast, or pounding heartbeats. These can occur at any time – active or resting – and can be felt in the throat, neck, and/or chest. If they are accompanied by chest discomfort/pain, fainting, shortness of breath, and/or severe dizziness, then seek emergency medical attention.

Contraindications and Indications

Before performing an exercise test, you must first identify your client's indications/contraindications. In medicine or fitness, indications and contraindications are very important when determining risk factors that could put your client in an unsafe environment.

An **indication** is a valid reason to use certain tests, medications, procedures, etc.

The opposite are **contraindications**: conditions or factors requiring the withholding of certain medical treatments or tests.

Contraindications to Exercise Testing

These are things to look out for *before* beginning a test. Absolute contraindications demand that, under no circumstances, should the test be performed. Relative contraindications call for concern; however the test may still be performed, though sometimes with modifications.

Absolute

- Acute myocardial infarction (within 2 days).
- Unstable angina, not previously stabilized by medical therapy.
- Uncontrolled cardiac arrhythmias, causing symptoms or hemodynamic compromise.
- Symptomatic severe aortic stenosis. – opening of the aortic valve is narrowed
- Uncontrolled symptomatic heart failure.
- Acute pulmonary embolus or pulmonary infarction. (any detached, traveling intravascular mass carried by circulation)
- Acute myocarditis or pericarditis.
- Acute aortic dissection.
- Suspected or known dissection aneurysm. (balloon-like bulge in an artery)
- Acute system infection, accompanied by fever, body aches, or swollen lymph glands.

Relative

- Left main coronary stenosis.
- Moderate stenotic valvular heart disease.
- Electrolyte abnormalities, such as hypokalemia or hypomagnesaemia.
- Severe arterial hypertension (greater than 200 mmHg and/or diastolic BP greater than 110 mmHg at rest).
- Tachyarrhythmias or bradyarrhythmias.
- Hypertrophic cardiomyopathy and/or other forms of outflow tract obstruction.
- Neuromuscular, musculoskeletal, or rheumatoid disorders that could be exacerbated by exercise. Symptoms can include: high sensitivity to hot or cold temperatures; lower extremity muscle weakness; foot drop; loss of sensation and/or balance/coordination; and tremors of varying degrees
- Ventricular aneurysm.
- Uncontrolled metabolic disease, such as diabetes, thyrotoxicosis, or myxedema.
- Chronic infectious diseases such as mononucleosis, hepatitis, or AIDS.
- Mental or physical impairment leading to inability to exercise adequately.
- High-degree atrioventricular block.

Absolute Indications

During testing, if any of these indications are seen, immediately terminate the testing.

- Suspicion of a myocardial infarction or acute myocardial infarction (heart attack).
- Onset of moderate-to-severe angina (chest pain).
- Drop in systolic blood pressure (SBP) below standing resting pressure, or drop in SBP with increasing workload accompanied by signs or symptoms.
- Signs of poor perfusion (circulation or blood flow), including pallor (pale appearance to the skin), cyanosis (bluish discoloration), or cold and clammy skin.
- Severe or unusual shortness of breath.
- CNS (central nervous system) symptoms such as ataxia (failure of muscular coordination), vertigo (an illusion of dizzying movement), visual or gait (pattern of walking or running) problems, and/or confusion).
- Serious arrhythmias (abnormal heart rhythms) such as second or third degree AV block, atrial fibrillation with fast ventricular response, increasing premature ventricular contractions, or sustained ventricular tachycardia)
- Technical inability to monitor the ECG.
- Patient's request to stop.

Relative Indications

These indicate that special attention ought to be paid to the exercise testing, to look for increasing reasons to halt the test. Like red flags, they bring attention to the specific problem. However, unlike *absolute* indications, they do not call for the immediate termination of the test.

- Increasing chest pain.
- Physical or verbal manifestations of shortness of breath or severe fatigue.
- Wheezing.
- Leg cramps or intermittent claudication (grade 3 on a 4-point scale).
- Hypertensive response (SBP >260 mm Hg; DBP>115 mm Hg).

- Pronounced ECG changes from baseline 1>2 mm of horizontal or down sloping ST-segment depression, or >2 mm of ST-segment elevation (except in a VR).
- Exercise-induced bundle branch block that cannot be distinguished from ventricular tachycardia.
- Less-serious arrhythmias such as supraventricular tachycardia.

Fitness Assessment: Five Components of Fitness

Once you have appropriately gauged the indications/contraindications/risk factors for your client, you may begin (with the clearance of a physician, when necessary) the fitness assessment. As stated before, the fitness assessment is comprised of **five components of fitness**: Cardiovascular Endurance; Muscular Strength; Muscular Endurance; Flexibility; and Body Composition.

Cardiovascular Endurance

Cardiovascular endurance (fitness), or cardiorespiratory fitness, is often considered the most important aspect of a client's total fitness; the ability to perform large-muscle dynamic, moderate-to-high intensity exercise for prolonged periods depends upon cardiovascular fitness.

A measure of the heart's ability to pump oxygen-rich blood to all the working muscles in the human body is one way to gauge cardiovascular fitness. If the heart is kept healthy, then the risk of numerous health problems is significantly reduced.

Low cardiovascular fitness in individuals markedly increases the risk of premature death by all causes, especially cardiovascular disease.

There are many ways of measuring cardiovascular endurance, from VO2 Max tests, to the Bruce test. We'll detail some of the more commonly-used ones here.

ECG

Cardiovascular Endurance can be measured in a hospital setting, where a physician monitors an exercise (stress) test (GXT) using an **electrocardiogram** (ECG) to evaluate heart rate, blood pressure, ventilation, and oxygen uptake responses during exercise. We've included a separate chapter for an in-depth look into ECGs.

Three-Minute Step Test

A less-expensive testing method, this can be given to healthy individuals wanting to begin an aerobic exercise program. Designed to measure cardiovascular endurance, this test is based upon how quickly the heart rate returns to normal after exercise.

Using a 12-inch high bench (or a similar-sized stair step), have the client step on and off for three minutes: up with first one foot, then the other; and then down with one foot, followed by the other. Encourage them to maintain a steady four-beat cycle – this is made easier if they are made to repeat "up, up, down, down." At the end of three minutes, have them sit down on the step or a chair. Immediately check their heart rate by taking their pulse for one full minute. The following charts detail the test interpretation:[3]

[3] Information can be found at http://www.topendsports.com/testing/tests/home-step.htm.

Three-Minute Step Test (Men) - Heart Rate

Age	18-25	26-35	36-45	46-55	56-65	65+
Excellent	<79	<81	<83	<87	<86	<88
Good	79-89	81-89	83-96	87-97	86-97	88-96
Above Average	90-99	90-99	97-103	98-105	98-103	97-103
Average	100-105	100-107	104-112	106-116	104-112	104-113
Below Average	106-116	108-117	113-119	117-122	113-120	114-120
Poor	117-128	118-128	120-130	123-132	121-129	121-130
Very Poor	>128	>128	>130	>132	>129	>130

Three-Minute Step Test (Women) - Heart Rate

Age	18-25	26-35	36-45	46-55	56-65	65+
Excellent	<85	<88	<90	<94	<95	<90
Good	85-98	88-99	90-102	94-104	95-104	90-102
Above Average	99-108	100-111	103-110	105-115	105-112	103-115
Average	109-117	112-119	111-118	116-120	113-118	116-122
Below Average	118-126	120-126	119-128	121-129	119-128	123-128
Poor	127-140	127-138	129-140	130-135	129-139	129-134
Very Poor	>140	>138	>140	>135	>139	>134

Bruce Protocol

The most widely – and internationally – used protocol for graded exercise testing is the **Bruce Protocol**[4] (or treadmill) test, which is a great indicator of **functional capacity** (how much the heart works, and how much oxygen one consumes). To record heart rate, ECG leads are placed on the chest wall.

- **Target Population**: Patients with suspected coronary heart disease; athletes who participate in sports with an emphasis on aerobic endurance; individuals who have mentioned experiencing chest pain, difficulty breathing, accelerated heart rate, etc.

- **Advantages**: Provides a measurement of maximum heart rate, information which is essential to setting the intensity of exercise programs.

- **Disadvantages**: Lengthy time requirements; large costs; requires a trained specialist to interpret ECG traces.

The test typically begins by running at an incline or gradient of 10%, speed 2.74 km/h. Every three minutes, the incline and speed of the treadmill will increase. Each level will see a 2% increase, as shown on the following chart:

[4] Have medical assistance, or test modifications, ready for those individuals with health problems, injuries, or low fitness levels.

Levels of the Bruce Protocol Test

Min.	Level	Incline	Speed	Speed	Gradient
3	1	10%	2.74 km/h	1.7 mph	10
6	2	12%	4.02 km/h	2.5 mph	12
9	3	14%	5.47 km/h	3.4 mph	14
12	4	16%	6.76 km/h	4.2 mph	16
15	5	18%	8.05 km/h	5.0 mph	18
18	6	20%	8.85 km/h	5.5 mph	20
21	7	22%	9.65 km/h	6.0 mph	22
24	8	24%	10.46 km/h	6.5 mph	24
27	9	26%	11.26 km/h	7.0 mph	26
	10	28%	12.07 km/h	7.5 mph	28

The Bruce Protocol Treadmill test measures maximal fitness, and so the individual will run/walk until they tire, with the result looking at the maximum time spent running (in minutes).

Formula for Estimating VO2 Max (Maximal Oxygen Intake):
Maximal Oxygen Intake (VO2 max) is a measure of cardiorespiratory fitness. It is a product of maximal cardiac output and arterial–venous oxygen difference. It is measured through an open circuit spirometer. Naturally, you may encounter patients who do not fit easily into each category. Do your best with a similar population, and choose which one best suits your needs.

T = Total time on the treadmill, measured as a fraction of a minute.
(i.e., A test time of 9 minutes and 30 seconds would be written as "T = 9.5.")

General:

$$\text{VO2 max} = 14.76 - (1.379 * T) + (0.451 * T^2) - (0.012 * T^3).$$

For Women:

$$\text{VO2 max} = 4.38 * T - 3.9.$$

\- or -

$$\text{VO2 max} = 2.94 * T + 3.74.$$

For Young Men:

$$\text{VO2 max} = 2.94 * T - 3.9.$$

For Men:

$$\text{VO2 max} = 2.94 * T + 7.65.$$

For those individuals that cannot walk or run on a treadmill, diagnostic testing through chemical tests is also an option. Persantine, Lexiscan TM, and dobutamine are some such chemical tests which allow for myocardial perfusion imaging.

Individuals with neuromuscular disorders who still require assessments for functional capacity and other such measurements can utilize the **cycle ergometer**, which is a low-impact machine. For those without leg performance, **arm ergometers** are another option.

Muscular Strength and Endurance

The ability to exert maximal force (using maximum or near maximum resistance) during limited repetitions is defined as **muscular strength**. When focusing on strength improvements, people generally work to increase their power and muscle mass, with gains in muscular endurance being secondary. Generated force is specific to the muscles involved, as well as the type, speed, and joint angle of the contraction.

Isotonic Contraction: Contraction wherein the muscle remains unchanged, and the distance between the origin and insertion shortens.

Isometric: Muscle contraction without shortening or change in distance between the origin and insertion.

[5]

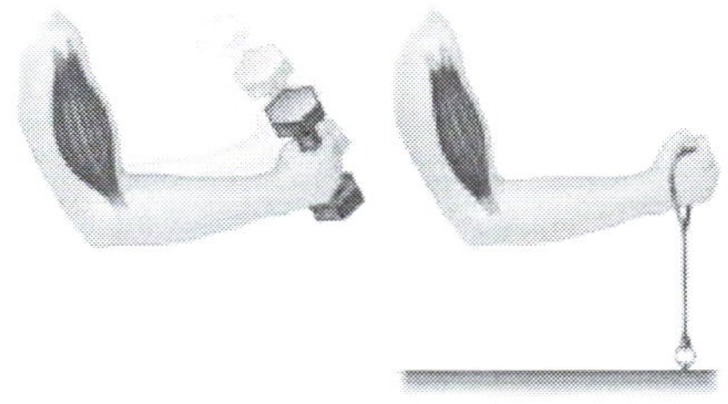

Eccentric vs. Concentric

When the muscle shortens to move the load, the isometric contraction is considered **concentric**; whereas muscles are **eccentric** when they are lengthening during contraction.

For example, consider a bicep curl exercise. **Concentric**: On the upward curl, the brachialis and the biceps branch shorten, pulling up the forearm with the weight. **Eccentric**: Now, if the weight was too heavy and began to fall, then the brachialis and biceps muscles would still be contracting (trying to hold up the weight) while lengthening.

Isokinetic: Pertains to the concentric (shortening) muscle or eccentric (lengthening) muscle, in which the speed and tension are constant throughout the range of lengthening or contracting.

Muscular strength tests are typically expressed in terms of how much weight can be lifted.

1RM Testing

This test measures the heaviest weight which can be lifted under the maintenance of good form, and is considered the gold standard for evaluating dynamic strength. The following are the typical steps for 1RM testing:

1. Once the client is familiarized with the necessary movement, have them undergo a light warm-up of 5 – 10 reps at 40 – 60% (light-to-moderate exertion) of their perceived maximum resistance.

[5] Isotonic *(A)* and Isometric *(B)* contraction.

2. Instruct the client to first rest for 1 minute of light stretching, and then to perform 3 – 5 reps at 60 – 80% (moderate to heavy exertion) of perceived maximum resistance.

3. Add 5 – to pounds. If the client successfully lifts that weight, allow a rest period of 5 – 10 minutes before adding another 5 – 10 pounds. Repeat until client cannot lift the adjusted weight. Record the last successfully completed lift as the 1RM.

4. To express the results relative to the client's weight, divide the 1RM by their body weight.

Handgrip Dynamometer

Also called the "Grip Strength Test," this tracks the development of a client's grip strength. The following are the typical steps for Handgrip Testing:

1. Have the client grip the dynamometer with their dominant hand, and apply as much pressure as possible.

2. Record the maximum reading (kg).

3. Repeat three times, using the highest value to assess the client's performance based upon the normative data for the grip strength test.

National Norms for 16 to 19 Year Olds[6]

	Excellent	Good	Average	Fair	Poor
Male	> 56	51 – 56	45 – 50	39 – 44	< 39
Female	> 36	31 – 36	25 – 30	19 – 24	< 19

Muscular endurance, on the other hand, is the ability to exert sub-maximal force (using less than maximum resistance) during repeated repetitions. When focusing on endurance improvements, people generally work towards increasing their muscle's ability to work over a period of time, with gains in power and muscle mass being secondary. During muscular endurance testing, it is important to not allow any rest periods between repetitions.

Partial Curl-Up Test

1. The client assumes the following position: supine on a mat, low back flat, knees bent at a 90-degree angle, arms at the side with palms facing down, middle finger of each hand touching a piece of tape placed next to the body. A second piece of tape is placed 10 centimeters beyond the first piece.

2. Set a metronome to the count of 50 bpm. (Metronomes encourage controlled movement; if one is unavailable, count off at the client's pace.) Have the client move through the range of motion, curling up to touch the second piece of tape before returning to the first in a controlled manner to the metronome's beat. The trunk ought to make a 30-degree angle with the mat.

3. Client should perform as many curl-ups as possible without pause, up to a maximum of 25, for 1 minute.

---

[6] Found in "Physical Fitness and Fitness Testing," by B. Davis.

Push-Up Test

1. Starting position:
   - For Males: Standard "down" push-up position, with the toes as the pivotal point: hands shoulder-width apart, back straight, head up.
   - For Females: Modified "knee" push-up position: hands shoulder width apart, back straight, lower legs together and in contact with the mat, ankles plantar flexed, head up.
2. Have the client raise their body by straightening their arms, before returning to the starting position to touch their chin to the mat. The stomach should never touch the mat. (Both Males and Females: Keep back straight at all times. Push-up must be to a straight-arm position.)
3. Count the maximal number of push-ups performed in good form. Stop when the client cannot maintain good form on two consecutive reps, or strains forcibly and cannot continue.

Body Composition

Bodies are made up of varying amounts of water, proteins, minerals, and fat. Assessing body composition can determine the amount of fat, bone and muscle in an individual's body. In the human body, muscle tissue takes up less space than fat tissue, but weighs significantly more. Therefore, body composition and weight combined determine the leanness and fitness of an individual. We'll discuss body composition in greater detail in the "Nutrition and Weight Management" chapter.

BMI

A client's height and weight makes up their **body mass index**.

$$BMI = 703 * \frac{Weight\ (lbs)}{Height\ (in)^2}$$

Underweight	< 18
Normal Weight	18.5 – 24.9
Overweight	25 – 29.9
Obese	≥ 30

A BMI reading is not completely accurate, however, as it not consider factors such as body frame, age, or percent fat. Therefore, a patient's **body composition** (percent body fat) is often a more reliable way to classify body weight. For assessment procedures for body composition, see our chapter on "Nutrition and Weight Management."

Flexibility

A client's **flexibility** is his or her possible range of motion around a specific joint or series of articulations. The ability to move a joint through an adequate range of movement is important for daily activities, as well as sports performance. Without normal movement within a joint, a person may not be able to function normally. While lack of flexibility may not seem like a very severe problem, a constant tightness in the muscles due to not stretching can lead to muscle pain, stiffness, and even injury. Assessments help determine a person's risk for future pain and injury.

Sit and Reach Test
This is the most common way to measure lower back, hamstring length, and hip joint flexibility. However, it does not effectively measure the lower back's range of motion (ROM).

- **Equipment required:** Sit and reach box (or, a ruler used along with a step or box)

- **Procedure:** Have the client remove their shoes and sit on the floor with their legs stretched out straight ahead, soles of their feet placed flat against the box. Both knees should be locked and pressed flat to the floor – you may assist by holding them down. With the palms facing downwards, and the hands on top of each other or side-by-side, the client reaches forward along the measuring line as far as possible. Ensure that their hands remain at the same level: one not reaching more than the other. After some practice reaches, the client reaches out and holds position for one to two seconds while the distance is recorded. Make sure that there are no jerky movements.

- **Scoring:** The score is recorded to the nearest centimeter or half inch of the distance reached by the hand. Some test versions use the level of the feet as the zero mark, while others set the zero mark nine inches before the feet. One modified sit and reach test adjusts the zero mark according to the subject's arm and leg length. The following table provides a general guide for expected scores (in centimeters and inches) for adults, using zero at the level of the feet (otherwise, add 23centimeters or 9 inches).

Sit and Reach Test Scores

	Excellent	Above Average	Average	Below Average	Poor
Male	> 34	28 – 34	23 – 27	16 – 22	< 16
Female	> 37	33 – 36	29 – 32	23 – 28	< 23

Fitness Assessment: Physical Assessment and Laboratory Tests

A fitness assessment may also utilize physical and laboratory tests.

Resting heart rate
Resting Heart Rate (HR) is obtained at the **apical site** (over the heart, at the 5th intercostals) with a stethoscope. Palpitation of the apical pulse is the point of maximal pulse **(PMI)**. A normal resting HR is 60 – 80 bpm.

Resting blood pressure
Resting blood pressure (BP) can be taken when the patient is seated, supine, or standing. BP is notated as the maximal output (the **systolic** reading) over the minimum output **(diastolic)**. This notation is not a fraction, and cannot be reduced.

- **Normal BP**: Less than 120/80.

- **Pre-hypertensive**: 120-139/80-89.

- **Stage 1 hypertension (HTN)**: 140-159/90-99.

- **Stage 2 HTN**: Greater than 160/100.

Typical, though less-common, tests include:

- Evaluation of abdomen for bowel sounds, masses, and/or visceromegaly.

- Auscultation (listening with a stethoscope) of the lungs, with specific attention to the uniformity of breath sound in all areas (absence of rales [crackling or rattling], wheezes, and other breathing sounds). For audio examples of different auscultations, see http://www.easyauscultation.com/lung-sounds-reference-guide.aspx.

    - Rales: Crackles or rattles occur during the opening of small airways and alveoli which were collapsed by fluid, exudate, or lack of aeration during exhalation.

    - Wheezes: Wheezing occurs when some part of the respiratory tree is narrowed or obstructed, or when the respiratory airflow velocity is heightened.

- Check for the absence or presence of tendon xanthoma and skin xanthelasma.

- Test for orthopedic issues.

- Palpitate and inspect lower extremities to determine presence of edema and/or arterial pulses.

- Test for proper neurologic function, including reflexes and cognition.

Common Tests for Different Levels of Risk
Those requiring Laboratory Tests can be broken into three categories:

1. Those with low, moderate, and increased (but without known disease) risk. In these cases, the following tests are common:

    - Fasting serum total cholesterol, LDL cholesterol, HDL cholesterol, and triglycerides.

    - Fasting plasma glucose, especially for those older than 45, younger but still overweight, or those showing any two risk factors for Diabetes Mellitus.

    - A thyroid function screening evaluation is appropriate, especially if dyslipidemia is present.

2. High Risk patients, with a known or suspected cardiovascular disease: Here, all category-one blood tests are recommended, plus the following cardiovascular tests:

    - Resting electrocardiogram (ECG).

    - Catheterization.

    - Radionuclide or echocardiography studies.

    - A chest radiograph (if heart failure is present or suspected).

    - A comprehensive blood chemistry panel, and a complete blood count as indicated by history and physical examination.

3. Patients with pulmonary disease:

   - Chest radiograph.

   - Pulmonary function test (recommended for all smokers older than 45 years old, and any persons presenting with dyspnea).

   - A number of specialized pulmonary studies.

Additional Knowledge to Study

The following information covers those subjects which are necessary to understand during a health appraisal and/or exercise test.

Periodization Phases
Periodization is the process of varying a training program at regular time intervals to bring about optimal gains in physical performance. Adding periodization phases into your client's exercise improves their muscular endurance, strength, power, motor performance, and/or muscle hypertrophy.

Resistant-Training Methods and Examples:

Variable Resistant: A resistance that changes over the ROM when an isotonic contraction is used to move a load.

Plyometric Exercise: Also known as "jump training," this training technique was developed originally for Olympic athletes to increase muscular power and "explosiveness." Plyometrics condition the body with dynamic resistance exercises that rapidly stretch a muscle (eccentric phase) and then rapidly shorten it (concentric phase).

Hopping and jumping exercises, for example, subject the quadriceps to a stretch-shortening cycle that can increase strength and vertical jump, while reducing the force of impact the joints.

Plyometric training is often used to condition professional and amateur athletes, since the exercises mimic the motions used in sports such as skiing, tennis, football, basketball, volleyball, and boxing.

Test Your Knowledge: Health Appraisal and Fitness Exercise Testing

1. Explain a graded exercise test.
2. What form must be obtained by the patient/client prior to a test?
3. A patient has auscultating lung sounds, similar to a crackle. What could this mean?
4. Identify three types of metabolic diseases. obesity, diabetes mellitus I and II
5. Give three examples of signs and/or symptoms in individuals with a metabolic disease.
   WT gain, high blood sugar levels, sluggish behavior
6. Signs and symptoms prompted by exercise in individuals with a neuromuscular disease.
7. What is an appropriate exercise testing method for an individual with a neuromuscular disease?
8. List two absolute contraindications to an exercise test. patient's request to stop; technical inability to monitor the ECG
9. List four relative contraindications to an exercise test.
   ↑ chest pain
   wheezing
   leg cramps
   hypertensive response
10. How is maximal oxygen uptake measured?

Test Your Knowledge: Health Appraisal and Fitness Exercise Testing – Answers

1. This test measures functional capacity. The test will use an estimated VO2 max, unless the spirometer is used to get an actual VO2 max. Also, a test exceeding seven minutes indicates prognostic cardiovascular fitness value, due to the increased work capacity. The most basic, and most widely-used, exercise test is the Bruce Protocol treadmill test which increases speed and elevation every three minutes, with the patient walking or running until they are impeded by either exhaustion or a contraindication.

2. Informed Consent.

3. This indicates fluid in the lungs.

4. Obesity, Diabetes Mellitus I and II, thyroid disease, renal disease, and liver disease.

5. High blood sugar levels (sign of Diabetes Mellitus and obesity); shakiness and disorientation (symptoms of hypoglycemia); weight gain, sluggish behavior, and hair loss (indicative of hypothyroidism).

6. High sensitivity to hot or cold temperatures; lower extremity muscle weakness; foot drop; loss of sensation and/or balance/coordination; and tremors of varying degrees.

7. An appropriate test would be a low-impact machine, such as a cycle ergometer.

8. Any listed on page 26.

9. Any listed on page 27.

10. Maximal oxygen uptake (VO2 max) is a measure of cardiorespiratory fitness. It is a product of maximal cardiac output and arterial–venous oxygen difference. It is measured through an open circuit spirometer.

Chapter 3: Exercise Prescription and Programming

As you already know, exercise programs are beneficial and imperative for many reasons. They not only improve overall quality of life, but daily exercise or physical activity helps keep the heart in good health. Heart disease is a leading cause of death, and consistent exercise reduces risk for heart disease and helps to lower cholesterol and reduce the risk of osteoporosis, arthritis, Type II diabetes, and high blood pressure. Exercise is also a huge component for losing weight and creating lean muscle mass. Daily exercise and a healthy diet help with obesity (which continues to increase in Americans). Individuals feel good when they exercise, because it increases energy levels and metabolism, and it creates endorphins that help improve mood and decrease stress.

There are many different options for exercise programs, depending on what goals your clients are trying to accomplish. Some people just want to feel better, while others are on a mission to lose body fat and gain lean muscle mass. Other individuals are seeking exercise to help with a chronic disease or are training for a particular sport, such as running a marathon. Whatever their goals are, there is an exercise program that will fit all clients' needs.

Knowledge of Physical Activity Recommendations

There are many components of exercise programs that you need to be aware of as a health fitness professional. Many people think that exercise solely consists of walking, jogging, or some other comparable cardiovascular activity. Although cardiovascular exercise is a vital component of an exercise program, flexibility, balance, core, and resistance training are also important components of a well-balanced fitness program.

Moderate-intensity exercise can be characterized as putting enough demand on the body during aerobic exercise to increase heart rate and respiratory rates. Some examples include walking, mowing the yard, or climbing stairs. Vigorous-intensity exercises are more intense and cause an even greater increase in heart rate. Many people will find it hard to talk at this level of activity, and examples include running, biking, or playing an intense sport.

Basic Knowledge of Prescription Guidelines

It is recommended that adults participate in 150 minutes per week (that is 30 minutes a day, 5 times a week) of moderate intensity activity or 75 minutes per week of vigorous intensity activity. For basic fitness levels and guidelines, moderate intensity is preferred. If your clients want to challenge themselves or improve their fitness levels, then they can participate in more vigorous activities, as long as they are healthy and able to do so without placing themselves at high risk of injury.

Flexibility is an important, often overlooked, part of an exercise program. Stretching should be incorporated into a workout routine on a daily basis. If a client does not stretch every day, then it is absolutely essential that he or she does on days when working out. Flexibility techniques can be used in the warm-up and the cool-down.

There are many different types of resistance training programs, depending on what your clients' goals are. A client's primary goal may be to lose body fat, build strength, gain power, or achieve overall toning. As the trainer, you will adjust resistance training routines based on their goals and abilities. For now, we will look at some general resistance training guidelines. A resistance-training program should be performed at least 2 days a week for 45-60 minutes. It should consist of 3 sets of 12-15 repetitions with a 30 second rest interval between sets. The tempo should be moderate level and the number of exercises should range between 7 and 9.

Prescription Guideline Techniques for the Healthy Population
An exercise description depends on factors that include fitness levels, fitness goals, and orthopedic limitations, as well as time restraints, exercise preferences, and equipment availability. It is important to determine the frequency, intensity, volume, time (duration), and mode (type) of exercise that is best suited for each individual that you work with.

Intensity refers to the level of demand that an activity places on the body. It is typically measured by heart rate, METs, or VO2 max. Moderate intensity is preferred for general health requirements. Frequency refers to the number of activities you participate in over a certain time frame, usually measured by a week. For general health requirements, the ACSM suggests aerobic activity 3-5 times per week. If are exercising on consecutive days, alternate between two modes. Some examples of mode are running, cycling, strength training, etc. Duration is the length of time spent exercising. For general health requirements, the ACSM suggests 20-60 minutes of continuous activity. Volume of a workout includes the duration and frequency of the activity performed within the time frame allotted for that training process.

Cardiovascular Endurance
Cardiovascular endurance is the ability of the heart to provide oxygen to muscles during physical activity for a prolonged period of time. It is a crucial component of an exercise program. Cardiovascular training is an aerobic activity that has many benefits; it can decrease obesity, hypertension, type 2 diabetes, depression, as well as increase immunity, blood lipids, glucose tolerance, and a sense of well-being. Some moderate intensity activities include walking, slow jogging, using the stairs, etc. If and when your client is ready, some vigorous intensity activities are running, biking, attending an aerobics class, or playing a competitive sport.

An important part of cardiovascular training is one's VO2 max. This is the highest volume of oxygen a person can consume during exercise. Basically, it is a measurement to determine one's cardiovascular fitness. The higher ones VO2 max, the fitter an individual is. The average VO2 max for a sedentary adult is around 35 ml/kg/min, while an elite endurance athlete's average is 70 ml/kg/min. The good news is that an individual can improve their VO2 max by increasing their training volume and intensity.

The intensity of an individual's cardiovascular training is typically measured by his VO2 max. The heart is the most important muscle in the body, and cardiovascular endurance is essentially how strong the heart is; therefore, the higher an individual's cardiovascular levels are, the stronger his or her heart is.

The Karvonen Formula
The Karvonen formula helps determine an individual's heart rate zone. The formula involves the maximum heart rate and the resting heart rate for an individual. MHR (maximum heart rate) is the fastest rate at which an individual's heart will beat in one minute. The formula to determine an individual's MHR is 206.9 – (0.67 * age). To determine an individual's resting heart rate, RHR, have the individual take his or her pulse for 60 seconds upon first waking up. Then subtract that RHR from the individual's calculated MHR and multiply the answer by 65 % (low end of the heart rate zone) and by 85% (high end of the heart rate zone). Then add each of these number back to the RHR that was found; this range is the target heart zone for that individual.

An example of the Karvonen Formula:

You have a client, who is 25 years old, with a resting heart rate of 65.

206.9 – (0.67 * 25) = 190 (MHR)
190 – 65 (RHR) = 125
125 * .65 = 75
125 * .85 = 106

75 + 65 (RHR) = 140
106 + 65 (RHR) = 171

This client's heart rate zone ranges from 140 - 171.

A MET represents an individual's resting metabolism or oxygen uptake. METs are a measurement of cardiovascular fitness and are a way for you to measure the intensity of your workouts. It is very simple to calculate METs.

Women: 14.7 – (.13 * age) = target MET
Men: 14.7 – (.11 * age) = target MET

When an individual achieves or surpasses their target MET, they possess good to excellent cardiovascular fitness. Just as an individual's VO2 max has the ability to increase, so can one's MET levels.

Body Mass Index

BMI stands for body mass index. This is not a way to determine body fat, but rather a simple method to determine whether your client's weight is relative to their height. This method does not take a person's body fat or lean muscle mass into account. Studies show that obesity related health problems increase when BMI is greater than 25. BMI numbers related to obesity are as follows:

- Mild obesity equals a BMI of 25 - 30.
- Moderate obesity equals a BMI of 30 - 35.
- Severe obesity equals a BMI of 35 or higher.

Stages of Conditioning

Your goal as a personal trainer is to design an effective exercise program for your client. You do not want to throw your client into a routine that they (or their body) will not be able to handle, so there are many things to consider when designing an exercise program, including. The client's current level of health and health history, orthopedic concerns (injuries, pain), personal health goals, current level of fitness, and whether he or she has ever been involved in a workout program before.

A musculoskeletal system can be over-trained when it is deconditioned. This means individuals are at a higher risk for injury when their bodies are in a state of low physical fitness, which includes muscle imbalances, decreased flexibility, and loss of core and joint stability. In the first 6 months of training and conditioning, the focus should be on developing basic strength and endurance, flexibility, efficient connective and supportive systems, stabilization, proper movement patterns, and cardiovascular fitness.

Periodization is an important concept in conditioning.

- Linear periodization is a continual progression of increasing intensity. The amount of weight is increased as the repetitions are decreased. This type of periodization is good for beginners and intermediate levels.

- Alternation periodization involves alternating between volume and intensity. This is a good method for more advanced clients.

According to ACSM guidelines, the initial stage of conditioning consists of a 10 - 15 minute warm-up followed by a moderate intensity activity for 15 - 30 minutes with 40%- 60% of HRR, 3 - 4 days a week.

The improvement stage of conditioning consists of a warm-up of 10 - 15 minutes followed by an activity with 50% - 85% of HRR. Have clients begin by doing the activity for only 30 minutes, but increase the activity duration by 10% - 20% every week.

Continue increasing intensity levels by 5% - 10% every two weeks until the goal is reached. Once goals have been reached, it is important to maintain conditioning with different activities.

Flexibility

Flexibility is the normal extensibility of all soft tissues that allow the full range of motion for each joint. Many people overlook the importance of flexibility training, but it plays an important role in injury prevention. Flexibility can also decrease the occurrences of muscle imbalances, joint dysfunctions, and overuse injuries.

There are many different types of stretching, but the three we will focus on are static, ballistic, and PNF:

1. Static stretching is a very common technique used as a corrective measure. It is the process of passively taking a muscle to the point of tension and holding the stretch for 10 - 30 seconds. This type of stretch allows the muscles to relax due to autogenetic inhibition and provide for better elongation of the muscle.

2. Ballistic stretching consists of uncontrolled bouncing, jerking, bobbing, or pulsing to achieve greater range of motion. This technique is *not* a preferred stretching technique due to its possible risk of injury and soreness. When ballistic stretching is performed, the stretch causes muscles to contract, leading to possible tearing of the muscle fibers.

3. PNF stands for Proprioceptive Neuromuscular Facilitation. This type of stretching was designed for the rehabilitation of patients. The main goal of this technique is to facilitate muscle relaxation and a fuller range of motion.

Muscular Strength and Endurance

Strength training benefits everyone. It helps to reduce body fat, create lean muscle mass, and burn more overall calories throughout the day. A consistent strength training program can also decrease the symptoms of many chronic diseases, help develop stronger bones, reduce risk of injury, help to control weight, and assist in overall strength in daily activities.

What is the difference between muscular strength and muscular endurance? We'll go over this in more detail in later chapters, but for now – **Muscular strength** is the maximal amount of resistance that a muscle or a group of muscles can overcome. A training program should consist of a progressive approach, because muscles adapt quickly, so they need to consistently be challenged. **Muscular endurance** is the ability of a muscle or group of muscles to overcome a sub-maximal resistance several times, consecutively. Basically, this means that an individual can lift lighter weights with more repetitions. This type of training helps with stabilization during training and with posture throughout an individual's daily routine.

There are many different types of exercises and strength training systems. The use of a bench press is an example of an upper body strength training exercise. A squat is an example of a lower body strength training exercise. The strength training system that is implemented for an individual depends on that individual's goals and abilities, and it will most likely be changed throughout the course of training. Here is a brief overview of common strength training routines:

- Single-set: One set of each exercise.
- Multiple-set: A multiple number of sets (3 - 5) for each exercise.
- Pyramid: Increasing or decreasing the weight with each set.
- Superset: Performing two exercises (within the same muscle group) back to back.
- Circuit training: Series of exercises, back to back, with little rest.
- Split-routine: Training different body parts on different days (ex. Day 1: chest, shoulder and triceps; Day 2: back and biceps; Day 3: legs; hamstrings, gluteal, quads, and calves).
- Horizontal loading: Completing all sets of an exercise before moving on to the next exercise.
- Vertical loading: Completing one set of all exercises before beginning the second set.

Different Types of Exercise

For clients who have a goal of general performance and overall health and well-being, the focus should be cardiovascular activities, resistance training, and flexibility.

- Flexibility exercises (stretching) can be performed seven days a week or a minimum of 5 days a week.
- Cardiovascular activities such as riding a bike, walking, jogging, etc., should be performed 3 - 5 days a week, or for at least 150 minutes a week.
- Resistance training (muscular strength and endurance) should be performed 2 - 3 days a week for 45 - 60 minutes.

As stated previously, exercise programs may have to be altered based on clients' goals and capabilities.

Proper Breathing

Proper breathing technique is crucial during strength training and aerobic activities. Breathing is the process of moving air in and out of the body. Inspiration is moving air into the body (inhaling) and expiration is moving air out of the body (exhaling). When performing aerobic activity it is important to focus on breathing. As a trainer, you should teach your clients to breath diaphragmatically (through the stomach). Breathing dysfunction corresponds with kinetic chain dysfunction. If you notice a client being unable to switch from an altered breathing pattern to a proper breathing pattern, refer them to a health care professional.

When muscles contract concentrically, you typically want to inhale and when muscles contract eccentrically you will exhale. For example, when performing a bicep curl you will inhale on the way up (concentric movement) and exhale on the way down (eccentric movement).

One particular method for breathing is the **Valsalva maneuver**, which is an attempt to breathe through a closed airway (attempting to exhale through a closed mouth and plugged nose). It serves to aid medical examinations and equalizes pressure in the ears and sinuses during ambient pressure changes (ex: diving).

During the Valsalva maneuver, a patient should go through the following four phases of physiological response:

1. Initial pressure rise:

    - Pressure will increase inside the chest, forcing blood out of the pulmonary circulation and into the left atrium. This causes a mild rise in stroke volume.

2. Reduced venous return and compensation:

    - First 5 to 14 seconds: The pressure inside the chest will impede the return of systemic blood to the heart, reducing the output of the heart and decreasing stroke volume.

    - First 15 to 20 seconds: When stroke volume has fallen, blood vessels will reflexively constrict with some rise in pressure. However, cardiac output and blood flow to the body remain low, while the pulse rate increases.

3. Pressure release:

    - 20 to 23 seconds: When the pressure on the chest is released, the pulmonary vessels and the aorta re-expand, decreasing left ventricular return and an increasing aortic volume, which causes a further initial slight fall in stroke volume. Venous blood can once more enter the chest and the heart, and cardiac output begins to increase.

4. Return of cardiac output:

    - 24 seconds and onwards: Blood return to the heart is enhanced by the effect of entry of blood which had been held back, causing a rapid increase in cardiac output. The stroke volume usually rises above normal before returning to a normal level, and the return of blood pressure, the pulse rate returns to normal.

If a patient deviates from this response pattern, it is a good indication of abnormal heart function or abnormal autonomic nervous control of the heart.

Because the Valsalva maneuver can increase blood pressure and can be harmful to some people, a modified version is to have clients attempt to exhale when the glottis is tightly shut, allowing for testing of cardiac functions and nervous control of the heart, without forcing air in the **Eustachian** (ear canal) tubes.

Concentric and Eccentric Phases

There are three basic muscle actions: eccentric contractions, isometric contractions, and concentric contractions:

1. When a muscle contracts eccentrically, it is exerting less force than what is placed on it. This results in a lengthening of muscle fibers. This is the strongest action of the three muscle actions. In an eccentric movement the muscle is moving in the same direction as the resistance.

2. An isometric contraction consists of a muscle maintaining a certain length. There is no movement occurring in this contraction. It is the second strongest muscle action.

3. The third is a concentric contraction. When a muscle contracts concentrically, it results in a shortening of muscle fibers, and it is exerting more force than is being placed on it.

Calculations

Target heart rate is a percentage of the maximum heart rate that an individual's heart rate is targeted to stay between. There are three zones, and clients' goals and fitness levels will determine which zone they should be exercising in.

- Zone 1 is called the recovery zone. In this zone an individual's target heart rate will be at 40 -65% of his or her maximum heart rate. Remember, MHR is based on the VO2 max, which is found using the Karvonen formula.

- Zone 2 is referred to as the aerobic endurance zone, which occurs between 65 - 85% of MHR.

- Zone 3 is anything above 85% of an individual's MHR, and is referred to as the peak zone.

Knowledge of RPE

RPE, rated perceived exertion, is used to measure the intensity of an exercise. The scale runs from 0 - 10, with zero being the easiest level and ten being the most difficult. For example level 0 would represent one sitting on a couch and level 10 would represent how one would feel after a difficult activity such as playing an intense sport. The RPE should be determined based on the mode of exercise.

To achieve the full benefit of exercise, it is recommended for RPE to be between levels 3 and 4. The RPE scale is at the top of the next page.

The RPE Scale:

0= Nothing at all
1= Very light
2= Light
3= Moderate
4= Somewhat heavy
5= Heavy
6= Heavy
7= Very heavy
8= Very heavy
9= Very heavy
10= Extremely heavy

Development of an Exercise Program

A **well-developed exercise program** is vital to meeting the needs of participating clients. Exercise prescriptions must address the client's needs, interests, and limitations; and, perhaps most importantly, they must enhance health through disease prevention, producing a change in the personal health behavior of an individual with continuous physical activity.

When designing an appropriate exercise prescription, you need to take into account five essential components: **mode, intensity, duration, frequency, and progression.** (FITT)

1. **Mode**: The type of activity or exercise within which the client will participate.

2. **Frequency**: How often, per week, the client will be participating in each exercise or activity.

3. **Intensity**: How hard the client's body works during the activity. The health and fitness goals, as well as the current level of fitness, of the client will determine their ideal exercise intensity, which can be measured by **target heart rate, talk test** (maintaining the intensity of an exercise at which conversation is comfortable)**,** and the **rate of perceived exertion scale** (also referred to as the **Borg scale**, this can be found on page 51.

   The human body has a built-in system to measure exercise intensity – the heart. Heart rate will increase in proportion to the exercise's intensity. You can track and guide exercise intensity by calculating Target Heart Rate (THR) range.

   For moderate physical activity, a person's Target Heart Rate should be 50 – 70% of their maximum heart rate. A good estimate of person's maximum heart rate is 220 beats per minute (bpm), minus their age. However, this is an estimated value. Use with caution.

4. **Duration**: How the long the activity or exercise session will last.

5. **Progression**: Changing your client's workouts to be effective and challenging.

When designing an exercise program, a health fitness professional should monitor the client's progress, keeping records of the client's adaption. The program should be dynamic, growing as the client adapts, in order to maintain exercise **consistency**, which helps achieve ongoing fitness results. Commitment to a regular workout regimen increases fitness level, improves health, and generates a greater sense of mental well-being.

There are four exercise principles of which a health fitness professional should have a good understanding before designing an exercise program for their client. They are: **specificity, overload, adaptation, and progression**.

The Specificity Principle

Exercising a certain body part, or a component of the body, develops *primarily* that part. Therefore, in order to become better at a particular exercise or skill, that exercise or skill must be exercised. A runner should train by running, a swimmer by swimming, and a cyclist by cycling. While having a good fitness base by undergoing general conditioning routines is helpful, if a client needs or wishes to be skilled in one particular area, then their prescription needs to include training specifically for that area.

The Adaptation Principle

The body has a fantastic ability to adjust to increased or decreased physical demands. This allows people to learn muscle coordination and develop sports-specific skills, such as batting, swimming freestyle, or shooting free throws. Practicing a skill or activity repeatedly makes it second-nature, and therefore easier to perform. People new to exercise are often sore after beginning a new routine, but after repeating the exercise for weeks and months, they will have little – if any – muscle soreness. That's adaptation!

↓ soreness to a new exercise overtime

The Principle of Overload

Greater stress than normal is required for training adaptation to take place. What this means is that – in order to improve fitness, strength, or endurance – workload must be increased accordingly. (You cannot gain without doing work.)

In order for a muscle (including the heart) to increase strength, it must be gradually stressed by working against a load greater than it is used to. To increase endurance, muscles must work for a longer period of time than they are used to, or at a higher intensity.

The Principle of Progression

This implies that there is an optimal level of overload that should be achieved, and an optimal time frame for this overload to occur. A gradual and systematic increase of the workload over a period of time will result in fitness improvements, without risk of injury. If overload occurs too slowly, then improvement is unlikely; *however* overload that is increased too rapidly may result in injury or muscle damage. For example, the weekend athlete who exercises vigorously only on weekends violates the principle of progression and most likely will not see obvious fitness gains.

The Principle of Progression also stresses the need for proper rest and recovery. Continual stress on the body and constant overload will result in exhaustion and injury. You should not train hard all the time, as you'll risk overtraining and a decrease in fitness.

Exercise Testing

Exercise testing elicits the body's reaction to measured increases in acute exercise. The changes in heart rate, blood pressure, respiration, and perceived level of exercise provide data that permit quantitative estimation of cardiovascular conditioning and function.

By monitoring heart rate and blood pressure, and continually observing the ECG, one can detect changes in the hemodynamic response and ischemic type ECG ST segment depression; this can aid in the detection and classification of those disturbances in heart rhythm and conduction which are associated with exercise.

If you are working with a client with cardiovascular disease (CHD), exercise testing is much more involved than usual. To see how your client's heart responds to an increased exercise demand, their physician may recommend them to participate in a graded exercise test (GXT); this diagnostic exercise testing is usually performed in a hospital setting with a physician present. This test is very important when you have someone with CVD, or whom their physician expects to be developing CVD.

Special Populations

Chronic Diseases

Chronic diseases – such as diabetes, cancer, cardiovascular disease, chronic heart failure, and pulmonary disease – are the leading cause of mortality in the world. They are diseases of long duration, and are generally slow in progression. Chronic diseases do not resolve spontaneously, and are rarely cured completely. They are the most common and costly of all health problems, but they are also the most preventable.

Cardiovascular Disease (CVD)

CVD refers to any disease that affects the heart or blood vessels. CVD can increase the risk for heart attack, heart failure, sudden death, high blood pressure, stroke, and cardiac rhythm problems, thus resulting in both a decreased quality of life and a decreased life expectancy.

The causes of cardiovascular disease range from structural abnormalities to infection, inflammation, environmental responses, and/or genetics. However, it can also be prompted by an unhealthy lifestyle. In order to prevent CVD, one must adopt a healthy lifestyle by exercising, maintaining a healthy diet (including the limiting of fatty foods), avoiding smoking, and minimizing stress.

Preventable, or treatable, CVD risk factors include: high blood pressure, high cholesterol, excess weight, physical inactivity, smoking, diabetes, excessive alcohol consumption, illegal drug use, and stress. Unpreventable risks include: previous heart attack, a family member with heart disease, increasing age, gender, and race.

Atherosclerosis (plaque formation) refers to the amount of lipid (fat) deposits in the medium and large arteries of the body. With a sedentary lifestyle, a diet that involves a high intake of saturated fat, high blood pressure, smoking, and any other toxic agent to the body, the endothelial cells of the artery can become damaged. Lipoproteins are deposited at the damaged site of the artery, and plaque formation (atherosclerosis) begins. These deposits can eventually impede blood flow through the artery. Atherosclerosis can occur anywhere in the body; but when it occurs in the coronary (heart) arteries, it can increase risk for a heart attack.

> **Exercise training** is an ordinary treatment for cardiovascular disease today because of the known health benefits of conditioning and strengthening the heart. Exercise, or aerobic training, improves blood circulation in the heart, as well as oxygen delivery. Exercise training reduces body fat and blood pressure; lowers total cholesterol, triglycerides, and LDL (bad cholesterol); and increases HDL (good cholesterol).

The level of exercise which a client first engages in will vary with each individual's needs and abilities. However, it is important for you as a professional to always stress the importance of physical activity as a preventative of CVD.

Obesity

Obesity has been labeled a chronic disease by the Centers of Disease Control (CDC), and has become a major health concern for people of all ages; one in every three adults, and nearly one in every five young people aged 6 – 19, are obese. This chronic disease is one of the leading causes of Type II diabetes, heart disease, and stroke. Obesity, however, can be preventable.

Modifiable behaviors such as getting a sufficient amount of physical activity every day; and consuming a healthy diet that is rich in lean proteins (chicken with no skin, 100% ground turkey, and fish – all baked, grilled, broiled, or boiled), high in fruit and vegetables, and low in saturated fats. When lack of activity and a high intake of saturated fat cause an overweight body, a person is at a higher risk for cardiovascular disease.

Diabetes

Diabetes is characterized by **hyperglycemia** (elevated blood sugars). There are two common forms of diabetes: Type I and Type II.

Type I diabetes is an autoimmune disease wherein the insulin-producing beta cells of the pancreas are destroyed by the own body. The pancreas cannot produce insulin, making it necessary for the person to administer insulin for the rest of their life. Type I diabetes is treatable, and maintainable, but not preventative.

In **Type II** diabetes, insulin receptors become resistant to insulin, and blood glucose cannot readily move into the cells. This causes hyperglycemia. Diabetes, if not controlled, can increase the risk for many complications that affect the blood vessels and nerves, including: vision impairment, kidney disease, peripheral vascular disease, atherosclerosis, and hypertension. Type II diabetes can be prevented.

Developing some of these complications increases the risk for heart disease and stroke. Many people with Type II diabetes are relatively inactive and overweight (or even obese). The development of excessive abdominal fat can also be attributed to age, family history, and lifestyle choices. In today's society, with its growing obesity epidemic, Type II diabetes is rapidly developing in children. However, it can be managed just as obesity: through the intake of healthy foods, and the maintenance of a healthy diet.

The Importance of Exercise

Exercise provides many benefits to bodies with and without chronic diseases. Although exercise will not always prevent or cure chronic diseases, it should still be encouraged. Exercise improves insulin sensitivity and reduces disease. Exercise protects against coronary artery disease, dyslipidemia (high cholesterol), hypertension, and obesity.

It can be difficult sometimes to exercise around a chronic disease – but there are always options. If you start working with a client with a chronic disease, both you and the client need open communication with the client's physician. You need to be sure the disease is stable before prescribing exercise.

Resistance Exercise vs. Aerobic Exercise

When the body has to use oxygen when exercising, it is undergoing **aerobic exercise**. Aerobic exercise is usually long in duration, but low in intensity, including such exercises as walking, biking, jogging, swimming, aerobic classes, and cross-country skiing. Aerobic exercise is different than resistance training, because aerobic exercise conditions the heart and lungs by increasing the oxygen available to the body; enabling the heart to use oxygen more efficiently. Aerobic exercise can decrease the risk for heart disease and stroke, due to its positive effects in decreasing blood lipid (cholesterol) levels and blood pressure.

Aerobic exercise has many other health benefits as well: reducing body fat, improving mood, reducing depression and anxiety, increasing energy, decreasing body tension, increasing sleep aid, and improving overall quality of life.

Aerobic Prescription

As with all exercise prescriptions, a clients' current health must be taken into account when designing a program. Take this case study:

> A client is moderately overweight, with no contraindications to exercise. He wishes to start exercising in order to improve his overall health. His goal is to exercise for 30 minutes a day, most days of the week.

In this example, a 12-week introductory plan is best to establish the habit of exercising in the client. Assign activities which are moderate in intensity; the best types would be those that use the large muscle groups (arms, trunk, legs), such as walking, a low-impact aerobics class, biking, swimming (if applicable), or light jogging.

All clients, regardless of their activity experience, should begin each exercise session with a brief warm-up: 5 – 10 minutes of light walking or biking, for example. Exercise sessions should also end with a cool-down period of 5 – 10 minutes.

Resistance exercise is defined as a movement performed against a specific opposing force, generated by resistance. Resistance exercise is also known as **strength training**, which causes the muscles to contract through such exercises as lifting weights, using resistance bands, pushups, pull-ups, lunges, and squats.

Resistance exercise is mostly known for improving physical appearance, but it also improves the body's overall health by contributing to weight loss. Resistance training increases the amount of calories burned during exercise and at rest. Your body uses calories all day long to maintain itself and support its various functions, such as digestion or breathing. The amount used for these purposes is referred to as the **resting metabolic rate**, which accounts for up to 75% of daily calories. Highly active tissue, like muscle, requires more calories to maintain, which means the more muscle you have, the higher your resting metabolic rate.

Resistance exercise also helps maximize bone mass, which reduces risk of osteoporosis later in life. Resistance training cannot reverse developed osteoporosis, , but it can help regenerate bone and slow loss, reducing risk of fracture. Additionally, muscle contraction during strength training exerts a pressure on the bone that increases bone strength and density.

Resistance training contributes to heart health by improving heart functioning; lowering blood pressure; and reducing levels of cholesterol, triglycerides, and blood sugar. During actual strength-training sessions, however, blood pressure can rise, making it potentially dangerous for those with high blood pressure. In those cases, lighter weights with more repetitions, rather than heavier weights with fewer, ought to be used. Consider consulting with other qualified professionals for guidance on a safe strength-training routine.

Resistance training can be accomplished with machines, free weights (barbells and dumbbells), or one's own body weight. Although many opt for machine-based workout sessions, which are easy to learn and perform properly, free weights offer some important advantages.

In general, all adults should perform 8 – 12 reps of 8 – 10 exercises on the chest, back, abs, shoulders, upper legs, lower legs, and arms at least **twice a week** for good health. Free weights, machines, or weight-bearing activities can provide resistance.

Adults 65 and older should strength-train 2 – 3 times a week, doing more reps with lighter weights.

However, creating an individual prescription is more complex; it must consider what exercises are most beneficial to the patient. Include the sequencing of exercises, the frequency of workouts, the **load** or weight, number of repetitions and sets, and the length of rest periods; these are based on training goals, progression, and variation.

With a client who is just beginning to exercise, it is important to monitor intensity and progress. A popular method of monitoring these factors is the Borg scale.

The Borg Scale

6	No exertion at all
7	Extremely light
8	
9	Very light
10	
11	Light
12	
13	Somewhat hard
14	
15	Hard (heavy)
16	
17	Very hard
18	
19	Extremely hard
20	Maximal exertion

[7]

[7] Image taken from http://www.home-health-care-physical-therapy.com/image-files/borgscale.jpg

Aerobic activities, like walking and cycling, should be done at level 13 (somewhat hard).

Strength activities, like lifting dumbbells and pushups, should be done at levels 15 – 17 (hard to very hard). Intensity can be increased as fitness increases. People often find that previously challenging activities become easier over time – those activities would then earn a lower score compared to that when they first started.

For example, slow walking on a treadmill may be a level 13 for your client in the beginning of their training. However, as fitness levels improve, it may be necessary to add an incline to the treadmill to get that same level-13 effort.

Acute and Chronic Adaptations

During exercise and long-term training, aerobic exercise and resistance training cause **acute** and **chronic adaptations** to occur in the body.

Acute adaptations occur immediately after, and sometimes during, exercise. Stroke volume and cardiac output are some examples of acute adaptations. **Stroke volume** refers to how much blood is ejected with each heartbeat. When aerobic exercise is performed, the venous blood that returns to your heart increases. This increases the amount of blood in the left ventricle that can be ejected throughout the body, increasing stroke volume.

Cardiac output is the product of stroke volume and heart rate. The amount of blood that your heart pumps per minute is increased during exercise, making this an acute adaptation.

An increased **respiratory response** (the amount of intake oxygen, as well as the amount of produced carbon dioxide) is also an acute adaptation to exercise. Carbon dioxide is a waste product of aerobic exercise that is expelled through exhalation. The body returns the deoxygenated blood to the lungs for gas exchange: CO_2 for fresh oxygen, or O_2. Because exercise demands more oxygen for the body, breathing rate increases in conjunction with heart rate to supply what is needed for energy metabolism.

Chronic Adaptations in the Heart

Acute responses during exercise often result in **chronic**, or long-term, adaptations to aerobic exercise, improving health and function. For example, a healthy cardiorespiratory will become more efficient at delivering larger quantities of oxygen to the working muscles. It would also promote a decrease in cardiovascular disease (CVD), stroke, high blood pressure, and obesity. These chronic cardiorespiratory adaptations are best developed through continuous and long-term interval training.

Chronic Adaptations in the Respiratory System

Aerobic exercise can also increase lung ventilation, where the lungs become more efficient. At rest, and during sub-maximal exercise, ventilation may be reduced due to improved oxygen extraction. However, during maximal workloads, ventilation increases in response to an increased tidal volume (amount of air breathed in and out in one breath) and respiratory frequency (the number of breaths taken per minute).

Pulmonary diffusion (the ability of the blood to extract oxygen from the alveoli) is also enhanced. These chronic adaptations occur over a period of time and can usually be seen as early as six weeks with aerobic training, but are more evident over twelve weeks of aerobic training.

Chronic Adaptations in the Muscles
Most people understand more about chronic muscular adaptations gained from resistance training (lifting weights, etc.). However, aerobic exercise aids the muscles as well.

After aerobic training, the muscles' oxygen utilization will increase. Aerobic training enhances the body's ability to first attract oxygen into the muscle cells, and then to utilize it to produce adenosine triphosphate (ATP) for muscle contraction and increased muscular fuel stores. This means that there is an increase in the muscular storage of glycogen, free fatty acids, and triglycerides, along with the oxidative enzymes required to metabolize these fuel stores and produce ATP.

Caloric Expenditures (Calories Burned)
Caloric expenditure depends on the amount of cardiovascular (aerobic) and strength (resistance) training one performs with each exercise, as well as the individual's metabolic rate (calories burned when the body is at rest). A person's metabolic rate accounts for up to 75% of the calories burned by the body each day to maintain normal body functions such as lung, heart, and brain function.

Aerobic exercise, resistance training, and exercise intensity all play significant roles in the amount of calories burned during an exercise session. Energy released from the breakdown of ATP – which itself is prompted by the contraction of muscles – fuels the contraction of *skeletal* muscle, which adds to the energy demands of the body; this raises caloric expenditure.

The **transport** and **consumption** of oxygen throughout the body during exercise are excellent health benefits for both cardiorespiratory fitness and weight loss.

At rest, the human body requires oxygen to keep all the vital organs of the body working properly; however, during exercise, the body demands and consumes significantly larger amounts of oxygen. The harder the body works, the more oxygen is needed to meet the demands of the working muscles.

This increased demand for oxygen during exercise, especially aerobic training, is part of what prompts weight loss. When sedentary people first start exercising, their bodies are not accustomed to the high demands of oxygen required to feed the working muscles. This is a reason why a sedentary person loses a lot of weight at the beginning of their exercise routine. However, as training continues over a period of time, the body begins to adapt to the demand of oxygen, becoming more efficient, without the need for as much oxygen as before they started training.

Important Note: We hear of **plateaus** in weight loss, where results seem to hold at a certain level. To continue losing weight, workouts must increase in difficulty. Increase either the work load or the program intensity so that the demand for oxygen consumption will continue to increase.

Cardiorespiratory fitness is also a benefit of oxygen transport and consumption. At the start of an exercise program, people begin to breathe more heavily in response to the heightened demand for oxygen. The heart pumps harder, increasing the oxygen uptake levels in the body, which in turn causes the lungs to work harder.

Prolonged physical activity therefore exercises more than just the targeted muscles; both the heart and lungs become stronger and more efficient.

There are many chronic adaptations in the heart with prolonged exercise, including but not limited to:

1. Red blood cells (hemoglobin) increasing in their oxygen-carrying capacity.
2. Cardiac muscle responding to aerobic training by increasing the size of the heart. This makes contractions more forceful, which in turn increases the amount of blood produced by each heartbeat.
3. Lower blood pressure.
4. Reduced blood lipids (lower levels of fat).

Factors to Consider When Prescribing an Exercise Program

The health fitness professional should understand environmental conditions when working with a client who has a chronic disease.

Changes in Temperature
When someone is exercising in **hot conditions**, extra stress is placed on the body; add that external heat to the increased core body temperature, and a person can risk serious illness when exercising in the heat. To cool one's body, the heart beats faster – and harder – to pump blood to the surface of the skin. It does this in order to assist with sweating, which is the body's attempt to cool itself. However, this leaves less blood for the muscles, and since the body utilizes the muscles during exercise, the heart again works harder to provide the necessary blood. Also, if humidity is high, the body faces added stress, because sweat doesn't readily evaporate from skin, pushing one's body temperature even higher.

Whenever temperatures reach 70 degrees Fahrenheit and the humidity is 70 percent or higher, the heart must work harder to cool the body. When the outdoor temperature climbs into the 80s (Fahrenheit) or beyond and there is high humidity, then the risk to health also rises.

If the body cannot cool itself enough, the heart experiences a high level of strain, leading to heat sicknesses. **Heat exhaustion** is a form of heat sickness that can lead to heat stroke. Symptoms of heat exhaustion include:

- Heavy sweating with cool, or clammy, skin.
- Fatigue.
- Nausea.
- Fainting.

Ultimately, if a person with heat exhaustion is not removed from the situation, then his or her organs can suffer damage – a potentially-fatal condition known as **heat stroke**.

Anyone can suffer heat stroke, but people with heart disease and other cardiovascular diseases are at greater risk. In those cases, the heart may not be able to perform the extra work demanded of it to maintain cooler body temperatures.

Some medications prescribed to patients with heart conditions reduce water in the bloodstream. These medications can reduce a person's ability to cool off in the heat. A health professional should note if a client has been prescribed diuretics or beta-blockers; if they have, then recommend that they ask their doctor about safe levels of water to drink in hot temperatures versus milder temperatures.

Other medicines decrease the amount of blood pumped by the heart (cardiac output) and limit blood flow to the skin, so the body is less able to cool itself by sweating. Other medicines can alter sense of thirst or increase the body's production of heat. If a client has a heart condition and is taking a medication that alters their heart rate, take extra precautions when designing their exercise program.

Heat stroke is an emergency. If a client ever experiences the following symptoms, advise them to apply cool water to their skin immediately and seek medical help.

Symptoms of Heat Stroke:

- High fever.
- Hot, dry skin without sweating.
- Pounding pulse.
- Dizziness.
- Nausea and/or vomiting.
- Confusion.
- Unconsciousness

If a client has heart disease, it is especially critical that they are told to avoid exercising when the temperature and the humidity are both high. For those cases, recommend that the client delays any intense exercise until the temperature has dropped and the humidity has reduced. Also consider prescribing physician-approved exercises wherein weather won't present an issue, such as indoor exercises or swimming.

On the other end of the spectrum, exercising in **cold conditions** can cause hypothermia: a decrease in body temperature wherein heat loss exceeds heat production and the body's temperature falls below normal. When temperatures drop, the heart has to work harder to help maintain your body's core temperature, and the added stress increases the risk of heart failure.

Some researchers think that cold weather may influence the human body in other ways (such as in hormones or blood vessel constriction) that also increase the likelihood of a heart attack or heart failure.

Because of these risks, extremely cold conditions are particularly dangerous for people with heart disease, as well as for babies and young children with complex congenital heart conditions.

Even if a client does not have a known heart disease, advise him or her to bundle up with layers, including a hat and gloves, when going outside. Recommend going slowly when shoveling snow or other physically challenging tasks. If a client does have a known heart disease, then the same warnings apply, to an even greater degree of importance. Before cold weather strikes, have the patient ask his or her doctor about safe levels of exposure to the cold, and which activities should be avoided.

Hypothermia and Heart Attack Symptoms
Hypothermia and heart attack are both medical emergencies. Instruct your client on the following, and if they suspect signs of either, tell them to **dial 9-1-1 immediately**.

Heart Attack Symptoms:

- Chest discomfort (Remember: not all people with heart attacks have chest pain.)
- Pain or discomfort in one or both arms, the back, neck, jaw, or stomach.
- Shortness of breath with or without chest discomfort.
- Breaking out in a cold sweat, or feeling nauseous or lightheaded.

Hypothermia Symptoms:

- Exhaustion or drowsiness.
- Shivering.
- Confusion.
- Memory loss.
- Fumbling hands.
- Slurred speech.

Exercising in a **high altitude** affects breathing rate, which can decrease the amount of oxygen into and out of the lungs. An increase in altitude decreases the partial pressure of oxygen, and reduces the amount of oxygen bound to hemoglobin (the protein in the blood that carries oxygen). As a result, the volume of oxygen carried in each liter of blood decreases.

Chronic obstructive pulmonary disease (COPD) refers to a group of lung diseases that block airflow upon exhalation, making it increasingly difficult to breathe. If a client has a chronic lung disease, such as COPD, breathing at even a normal altitude can be difficult. The higher the altitude, the less amount of oxygen they can inhale. Precautions should be taken when designing an exercise program for this client.

Wellness and Exercise Design

What is wellness?
Wellness and good health have historically been seen as freedoms from disease; therefore, a lack of illness equaled health. This historical perspective is changing; while virtually everyone agrees that absence from illness is a primary component of being healthy, it doesn’t indicate anything about your state of well-being.

As a state of health, wellness is closely linked to lifestyle. All individuals have a responsibility to themselves to provide for the essentials of good health – proper weight control, good nutrition, physical activity and exercise, and controlling health risk factors, such as tobacco, alcohol, and drug use and/or abuse.

Research studies related to wellness indicate that Americans who take good care of themselves and make healthy lifestyle choices are healthier, happier, more productive, miss less work, and have lower healthcare costs.

Much more than simply an absence of illness and/or disease, wellness is a proactive and preventative approach that is designed to provide optimum levels of health, emotional, and social functioning. It involves the recognition of psychological, physical, spiritual, and social needs; all of which are necessary for higher levels of functioning.

Wellness is a lifelong journey, from staying healthy to managing conditions.

Wellness strategies include anything from staying healthy, to getting healthy and managing ongoing health conditions. Quitting smoking after one finishes a pack of cigarettes is one strategy; another could be starting an exercise program on the first day of the month. Strategies are about making healthier goals and having an action plan to accomplish the wellness mission.

Many employers are now developing wellness strategies for their employees to adopt healthier lifestyles. By developing these strategies many employers can expect a $1 to $3 return on investment for preventive services and health promotion. Employee health affects more than just medical costs; a healthy workforce is a more productive workforce.

Exercise Programming

Programming guidelines are important to consider when developing a cardiorespiratory exercise program. ACSM recommends training at a moderate intensity at 55 – 69% of maximum heart rate, or high intensity at 70 – 89% of your maximum heart rate.

If a client is new to exercise, begin at 55% maximum heart rate, gradually increasing the intensity level as their fitness improves. Clients should always feel challenged, but not prohibitively so.

Cardiorespiratory Training

Each session should last between 20 and 60 minutes, three to five days per week. The longer clients train, the greater their training adaptive response will be, nut they should never overdo it! The body must rest in order to adapt and recover from the stress of training.

Muscular Training

Muscular strength and endurance is also an important component in designing an exercise program for your client. The ability to exert maximal force (using maximum or near maximum resistance) during limited repetitions is defined as **muscular strength**. When focusing on strength improvements, people generally work to increase their power and muscle mass, with gains in muscular endurance being secondary.

Muscular endurance, on the other hand, is the ability to exert sub-maximal force (using less than maximum resistance) during repeated repetitions. When focusing on endurance improvements, people generally work towards increasing their muscles' ability to work over a period of time, with gains in power and muscle mass being secondary.

ACSM Strength Training Recommendations

- When participating in a resistance training exercise program, ACSM recommends that you involve eight to ten exercises for the major muscles, with at least one set for each exercise.
- Eight to twelve repetitions per set of exercise on two or three nonconsecutive training days per week.
- Full-range movements which are pain-free.
- Moderate speed movements (approximately six seconds per repetition).[8]

A client's muscular strength and endurance program should begin using three exercise approaches: using their own body-weight, resistance machines, or free-weights. Ideally, all three will be worked into the program.

Body Weight

As the name suggests, these exercises utilize the body's weight as resistance. Exercises such as push-ups, sit-ups, jumping jacks, chin-ups, and leg lifts are well-suited for this type of program.

Advantage: These exercises can be performed just about anywhere, without the need for equipment.

Disadvantage: It is difficult to both increase the resistance easily and target specific muscle groups.

Resistance Machines

These exercises use specific machines which target certain muscles.

Advantage: These exercises allow your client to control resistance and isolate specific muscles.

Disadvantage: Requires special equipment.

Free-weights

These exercises depend upon using weights, such as dumb-bells or exercise bars, to perform repetitions.

Advantage: Client can control resistance, isolate specific muscles, and improve muscle balance using (at a minimum) a bench and some weights.

Disadvantage: Risk of injury is higher than with machine-weights, since the resistance is not mechanically supported.

When working in a fitness center, **weight room teaching skills** are essential in preventing injury and lawsuits. Exercise equipment can be dangerous if operated improperly; fingers can be smashed from

[8] Information can be found at pfswellness.com/.../ACSM_STRENGTH_TRAINING_GUIDELINES

the weights, and improper weight-lifting posture can be very damaging. Squats can cause knee pain, especially when they're performed incorrectly. Further, wear on knees from sports and other activities can make them more vulnerable to health conditions such as arthritis, which can exacerbate both pain and injuries. Learning to perform squats properly can help minimize discomfort and pain during the exercise. Therefore, a significant amount of time must be spent teaching a client how to perform all prescribed exercises safely.

Test Your Knowledge: Exercise Prescription and Programming

1. Which of the following is NOT a benefit of an exercise program?
   a) Decreased body fat.
   b) Decreased blood pressure.
   c) Increased risk of type 2 diabetes.
   d) Increased metabolism.

2. Exemplify the difference between moderate intensity exercise and vigorous intensity exercise.

3. The level of demand that an activity place on the body is:
   a) Resistance.
   b) Weight.
   c) Intensity
   d) Frequency.

4. The ACSM suggests what amount of time of continuous physical activity for general health requirements?

5. True/False: An individual can improve their VO2 max by increasing their training volume and intensity.

6. Determine a 30 year old client's target heart rate zone with a resting heart rate of 65.

7. ______________________ represents an individual's resting metabolism or oxygen uptake, and is a way for you to measure the intensity of your workouts.

8. What should your focus be in the first 6 months of training and condition?

9. True/False: Ballistic stretching is a popular technique. Why or why not?

10. True/False: Muscular endurance is the same thing as muscular strength.

11. When muscles are contracting concentrically an individual should:
   a) Inhale.
   b) Exhale.
   c) Hold his or her breath.
   d) None of the above.

12. A lengthening of the muscle fibers is what type of action?
   a) Isometric.
   b) Concentric.
   c) Flexibility.
   d) Eccentric.

13. Define the progression principle.

14. How often should children between ages 5 and 12 participate in exercise?
   a) Once a week.
   b) Every other day, for 3 hours at a time.
   c) Every day, for 60 minutes.
   d) Only when they request exercise.

15. List the five essential exercise components affecting the attainment of physical fitness.

16. True/False: Cardiovascular disease (CVD) is an abnormal function of the heart or blood vessels and lungs.

17. Which of the following is not an aerobic exercise?

a) Cross-country skiing.
b) Swimming.
c) Strength training.
d) Walking.

18. True/False: Chronic adaptions occur during an exercise session.

19. Which of the following is not a chronic disease?

a) Cardiovascular disease.
b) Pulmonary disease.
c) Diabetes.
d) Obesity.

20. True/False: Chronic diseases are diseases of long duration and generally slow in progression.

21. True/False: Many people with Type II diabetes are relatively inactive and overweight, or obese.

22. True/False: Exercise testing elicits the body's reaction to measured increases in acute exercise.

23. True/False: Aerobic exercise is usually short in duration, but high in intensity.

24. Which of the following is not defined as a resistance exercise?

a) Lunges.
b) Push-ups.
c) Swimming.
d) Bench press.

25. True/False: Exercising in a high altitude affects breathing rate, which increases the amount of oxygen into and out of the lungs.

26. Which of the following is not an absolute indication in exercise testing?

a) Suspicion of a myocardial infarction or acute myocardial infarction (heart attack).
b) Severe or unusual shortness of breath.
c) Any chest pain that is increasing.
d) Severe or unusual shortness of breath.

Test Your Knowledge: Exercise Prescription and Programming – Answers

1. **c)** Increased risk of Type 2 diabetes.
   Exercise keeps your heart in good health, decreases body fat, creates lean muscle mass, increases metabolism, reduces risk of osteoporosis, arthritis, type II diabetes, decreases blood pressure and cholesterol, and boosts self-esteem.

2. Moderate-intensity exercise puts enough demand on the body during aerobic exercise to increase heart rate and respiratory rates. Ex. Walking, climbing the stairs, mowing the yard.

   Vigorous-intensity exercise is more intense than moderate intensity exercise and causes an even greater increase in heart rate. Ex. Running, playing an intense sport.

3. **c)** Intensity.

4. 20 - 60 minutes.

5. **True**.

6. Target heart rate = 144 -168.

7. METs.

8. You should focus on developing basic strength and endurance, flexibility, efficient connective and supportive systems, stabilization, proper movement patterns, and cardiovascular fitness.

9. **False**. It is not popular due to the fact that it has a possible risk of injury and soreness.

10. **False**.

11. **a)** Inhale.

12. **d)** Eccentric.

13. The progression principle states that there is a desired level of overload that should be achieved in an optimal amount of time.

14. **c)** Every day, for 60 minutes.

15. **Mode, Frequency, Intensity, Duration,** and **Progression**.

16. **False**. Cardiovascular disease (CVD) is an abnormal function of the heart or blood vessels.

17. **c)** Strength training (the use of resistance for muscular contraction to build the strength, anaerobic endurance, and size of skeletal muscles).

18. **False**. Chronic adaptations occur with long-term aerobic and resistance training. They occur over a period of time and can usually be seen as early as 6 weeks.

19. d) Obesity.

20. True. Chronic diseases are diseases of long duration, generally slow in progression.

21. True. Many people with Type II diabetes are relatively inactive and overweight or obese, particularly with excessive abdominal fat.

22. True. Exercise testing elicits the body's reaction to measured increases in acute exercise.

23. False. Aerobic exercise is usually long in duration, but low in intensity.

24. c) Swimming (defined as an aerobic exercise).

25. False. Exercising in a high altitude affects breathing rate, which can decrease the amount of oxygen into and out of the lungs. An increase in altitude decreases the partial pressure of oxygen and reduces the amount of oxygen bound to hemoglobin (protein in the blood that carries oxygen).

26. c) Any increasing chest pain is a Relative Indication.

Chapter 4: Exercise Physiology and Related Exercise Science

Exercise Science covers a broad range of topics: physical activity, exercise, athletic performance, etc. Understanding how the body works is essential to providing safe and effective exercise prescriptions.

Bioenergetics

All movement within our body – in fact, every operation in our body – depends upon energy to function. **Bioenergetics** describes the processes of transferring energy from consumed foods throughout the body, supplying the contracting muscles with usable energy called adenosine triphosphate **(ATP).** This energy, or fuel, drives the body to operate.

ATP is necessary for all energy-requiring processes in cells. All muscle cells contain a small amount of ATP at all times, but that ATP is consumed almost immediately after exercise starts.

To replenish this energy, and maintain activity, ATP must be replenished via other energy pathways or energy systems.

Systems
There are three systems to know when covering bioenergetics:

1. **The Phosphagen System** is the body's energy system that uses immediate stored energy inside the muscle cell. This energy system is composed of ATP and phosphocreatine (PCr). Phosphocreatine and ATP are stored inside the muscles cells. Phosphocreatine is used for all-out effort and explosive power exercises like **sprinting** and **weightlifting**. The phosphocreatine system can sustain physical activity for no more than 30 seconds.

2. **The Nonoxidative System**, sometimes called the lactic acid or glycolytic system, is the body's short-term energy system. It allows ATP and phosphocreatine to be resynthesized at a rapid rate.

   This system is sometimes referred to as the **anaerobic** (without oxygen) pathway, because oxygen is not required for ATP production. Instead, this system uses carbohydrates (glucose and glycogen) for ATP production.

   The nonoxidative system is sometimes referred to as the **lactic acid system**, because lactic acid is produced when carbohydrates are broken down without the use of oxygen. Lactic acid, or lactate, accumulates in the muscles and contributes to muscle fatigue.

   The nonoxidative system is used for physical activities that require high-intensity effort. It provides energy to the working muscles during activities which last from 30 seconds to 3 minutes. These activities can be anything from running up the stairs to passing another participant in a race.

3. **The Oxidative System** is the body's long-term energy system. It breaks down carbohydrates (glucose and glycogen) *and* fats (lipids) from the foods in order to synthesize ATP. In this energy system, a very limited extent of proteins can be broken down into glucose as well, but proteins are not a preferred fuel source.

This system is also called the **aerobic** (with oxygen) pathway, because oxygen is required for this system to proceed. This system produces a large amount of ATP, unlike the Phosphagen system and the nonoxidative system.

The oxidative system's metabolic by-products are water and carbon dioxide. (Remember, the nonoxidative system's by-product: lactic acid.)

Unlike lactic acid, water and carbon dioxide do not cause the muscle to fatigue.

The oxidative system produces energy for those physical activities that last more than 3 minutes; as well as those activities where intensity is limited, like running a marathon or hiking.

While this system produces a larger amount of ATP than the other systems, it takes a longer time to produce that energy. Therefore, when the working muscle demands more than is being provided, the muscle will rely on the nonoxidative system for energy as well. This cooperation between the oxidative and nonoxidative systems is called the **anaerobic or lactate threshold**.

Blood

Blood has many functions, but its most important job is the transport of oxygen to working muscles, tissues, and organs.

Plasma
Plasma is the fluid part of the blood. Its main component is water (90 – 93%), but it also contains some proteins, electrolytes, gases, nutrients, waste products, and various hormones.

While plasma carries a small amount of oxygen, most of the body's oxygen is delivered through the cells of the blood.

Erythrocytes are red blood cells, and they contain a protein called **hemoglobin**. These are the most abundant types of cells in blood, accounting for more than 99% of the blood's cells. Oxygen is bound to hemoglobin for transportation; hemoglobin also carries some of the carbon dioxide (30%) in the body.

A **hematocrit** is a blood test that measures the amount of erythrocytes within the blood. The hematocrit levels are slightly higher in men than in woman, due to higher testosterone levels.

Leukocytes are white blood cells. They are the body's defense system, working to destroy any potentially infectious agents that enter the body.

Platelets are made up of many other parts of cells. They go wherever there is damage to the wall of a blood vessel to stop blood loss. If a body part is cut, platelets rush to the scene to clot the blood so that a person would not bleed out.

The Effects of Exercise on Blood
Hyperemia is the increased amount of blood flow to the working muscles of the body. As exercise increases, so too does the delivery of oxygen and nutrients to the muscles. This in turn increases the removal of waste products such as lactate and carbon dioxide.

Cardiovascular drift occurs when prolonged endurance exercise increases body temperature. To prevent overheating, plasma is moved from the blood vessels into the surrounding tissue. This provides the body with more water for sweating, which cools down the body. This drift can cause increased heart rate, because it decreases the total volume of blood and decreases the stroke volume.

In turn, the movement of plasma out of the blood leads to **hemoconcentration** – a decrease of fluids within the blood – which makes sense, since plasma is the fluid part of the blood. Hemoconcentration can lead to elevations in hematocrit and hemoglobin values.

Endurance training produces more erythrocytes (red blood cells), and therefore more hemoglobin, which increases the oxygen carrying capacity of blood to the working muscles. Training also prompts an increased plasma volume, which leads to a higher stroke volume and lower resting heart rate.

Anatomy and Physiology of Cardiovascular and Pulmonary Systems

The **pulmonary System** is divided into the upper and lower respiratory tracks.

The upper respiratory track consists of the nose, the pharynx (throat), and larynx (voice box).

The lower respiratory track consists of the trachea (wind pipe), lungs, bronchi, bronchioles (passage ways into the alveoli), and the alveoli (air sacs).

The human body has two lungs; these are organs that help us breath in air. The right lung has three lobes, and the left lung has two lobes. The lungs occupy pleural cavities that are covered by a **pleural membrane**. The pleural membrane helps separate the two lungs from each other.

The **apex**, the top of each lung, extends into the base of the neck above the first rib. Each lung has a **base** as well, which rests on the diaphragm.

The **diaphragm** is a respiratory muscle that allows us to breath. It is dome-shaped, and it separates the abdominal cavity (stomach) from the thoracic cavity (chest). This muscle contracts and relaxes as we breathe.

As we breathe through our nose and mouth, air will pass through the pharynx and larynx and down through the cartilage-lined trachea into our lungs. Air then passes through the bronchiole tubes into a cluster of **alveoli**. Alveoli are air sacs that exchange gases (oxygen and carbon dioxide) between our lungs and the blood.

Inhalation causes the diaphragm to move downward; the intercostal muscles (muscles between the ribs) then pull the ribcage up, therefore enlarging the thoracic (chest) cavity.

Exhalation causes the diaphragm to move upward. Now the intercostal muscles relax, causing less pressure inside the thoracic cavity. However, there is an increased pressure inside the lungs, which causes air to be expelled through the nose and mouth.

Trachea

Another name for the trachea is the wind pipe. It is made up of C-shaped cartilage rings that serve three important functions:

1. The C-shaped cartilage rings offer support for the trachea. They support, protect, and maintain an open airway.

2. The tough cartilage prevents overexpansion of the respiratory system.

3. The trachea lies anterior to the esophagus; it supports the esophagus, and allows for large amounts of food to pass down into the stomach by collapsing slightly.

Assessing the carotid and radial pulses

Heart rate, called a **pulse** due to the pulsating feeling in the blood vessels near the skin, can be measured on any large or medium-sized artery. Gentle compression of the artery by the index and middle finger together allows for the detection of a pulse. The two most common arteries that are assessed are the carotid artery (in the neck) and the radial artery (in the wrist). [9]

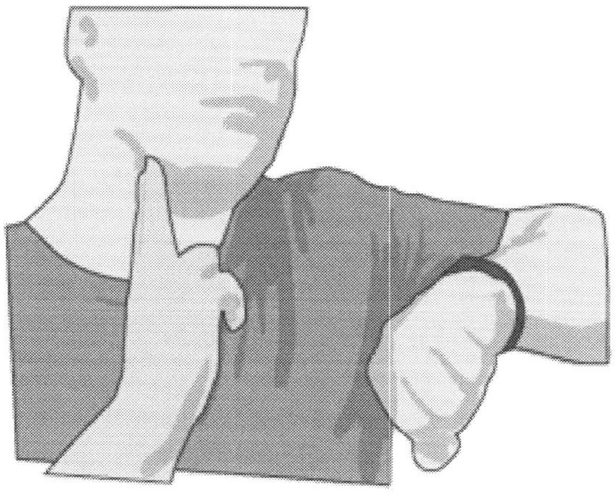

The **carotid artery** is divided into the left and right carotid, and lies on each side of the neck. It runs along the side of the trachea (windpipe) and below the mandible (jaw bone).

To assess the carotid pulse, place index and middle finger below the jaw and the side of the neck. Hold fingers together and press gently; move fingers around until pulse is felt.

Count the number of times the pulse is felt in 10 seconds using a second hand watch. Multiply this number by six to find the amount of heart beats in one minute.

The **radial artery** branches off the brachial artery (major blood vessel of the upper arm) and runs towards the thumb along the forearm.

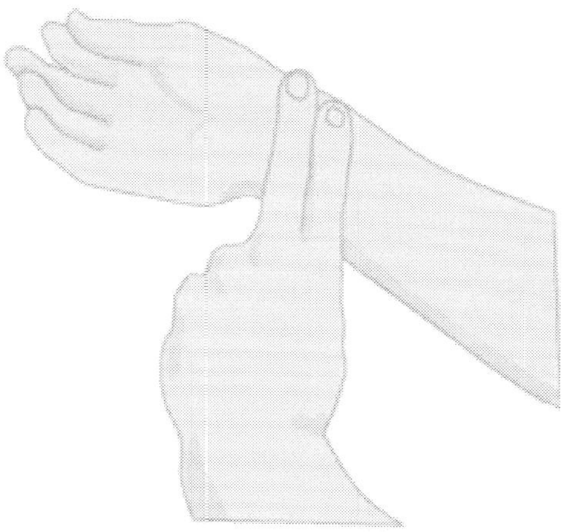

To assess pulse, place index and middle finger together and press gently on the thumb side of the wrist until pulse is felt. If no pulse is felt, move fingers around until pulse is felt.

Count the number of times the pulse is felt in 10 seconds, and multiply that by six to find the amount of heart beats in one minute.

---

[*] Images taken from: http://www.topendsports.com/testing/heart-rate-measure.htm Measuring heart rate-1997-2000. All rights reserved.

The **Cardiovascular System** consists of the heart, as well as two networks of blood vessels called the **pulmonary** and **systemic** circulatory systems.

1. **Pulmonary Circulation**: The part of the cardiovascular system that works with the lungs. The right atrium in the heart receives oxygen-depleted blood from the body. The heart then pumps oxygen-depleted blood into the lungs to be re-oxygenated. The left atrium receives that oxygenated blood from the lungs.

2. **Systemic Circulation**: The part of the cardiovascular system that circulates blood to all parts of the body, except for the lungs. It transports oxygenated blood away from the heart and carries oxygen-depleted blood back towards the heart.

Anatomy of the Heart

For a detailed image of the heart, see page 71.

The heart is a very complex system made up of four chambers, four valves, and multiple blood vessels.

The **four chambers** are the right atria, the left atria, the right ventricle, and the left ventricle.

Inside the ventricles are the four valves:

1. **Tricuspid Valve**: Located between the right atrium and the right ventricle.

2. **Bicuspid (mitral) Valve**: Located between the left atrium and left ventricle.

3. **Pulmonic Valve**: Located between the right ventricle and pulmonary artery.

4. **Aortic Valve**: Located between the left ventricle and the aorta.

Valves regulate the pressure inside the ventricles and prevent backflow. As blood fills the ventricles, the valves start to close; this builds up pressure. When the pressure is very high, the ventricle will contract and squeeze out the blood forcefully, either into the lungs or out of the aorta to the rest of the body.

The heart is connected to the rest of the body through a series of blood vessels. These are: **arteries**, **arterioles**, **capillaries**, **venules**, and **veins**.

Arteries are large blood vessels. They carry oxygenated blood away from the heart. To remember this, associate the "a" in "artery" with the "away." (**A**rteries carry blood **a**way from the heart.)

Arteries branch into smaller arteries called **arterioles**, which in turn branch off to form **capillaries**. Capillaries are extremely small, and they allow for the exchange of nutrients and gases within the tissue.

As these exchanges take place, several capillaries will join to form **venules**. Venules return oxygen-depleted blood back towards heart.

Just as the larger arteries grew smaller the further away from the heart they went, so too do the venules grow larger as they return to the heart. A number of venules form the larger blood vessels called **veins**.

Veins create more pressure inside the blood vessel, which helps return oxygen-depleted blood back to the heart.

The following chart illustrates the flow of blood through the heart.

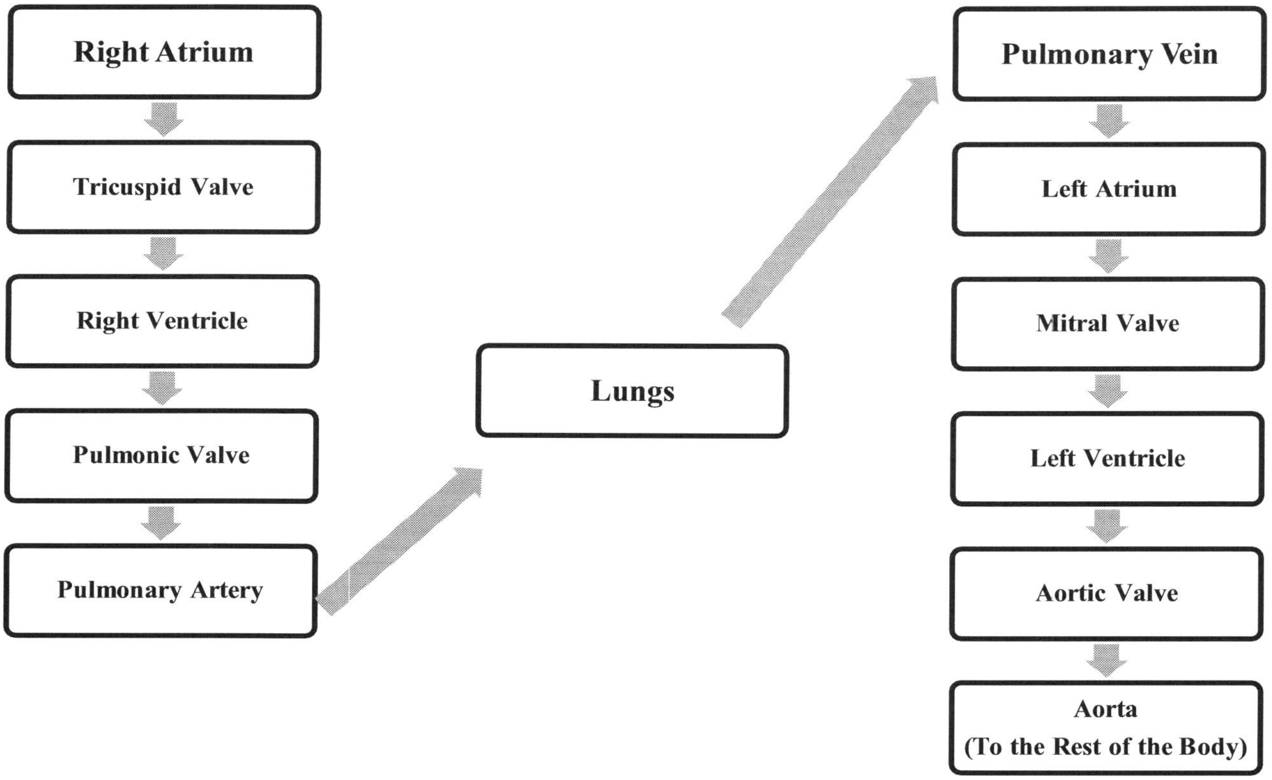

Oxygen-depleted blood is returned to the heart through the **inferior vena cava** (large vein that carries oxygen-depleted blood into the heart from the lower half of the body) or the **superior vena cava** (large vein that carries oxygen-depleted blood from the upper half of the body).

Blood enters the right atrium. The blood flows through the tricuspid valve into the right ventricle.

After the blood finishes filling the right ventricle, the tricuspid valve closes to allow pressure build up and to prevent blood from flowing back into the right atrium.

The right ventricle will then forcefully squeeze the blood through the pulmonic valve into the pulmonary artery; the pulmonary artery takes the blood away from the heart and into the lungs.

Inside the lungs, gases are exchanged. Oxygenated blood is picked up and returned to the heart via the pulmonary vein. From the pulmonary vein, blood enters the left atrium and then flow through the mitral valve (also called the bicuspid valve) into the left ventricle.

After the left ventricle is filled, the mitral valve closes to allow pressure build up and to prevent blood from flowing back into the left atrium.

Pressure builds up due to the closed bicuspid (mitral) valve, and, after enough pressure is built up inside the left ventricle, oxygenated blood will be forcefully expelled through the aortic valve into the aorta.

The aortic valve prevents blood from flowing back into the left ventricle. Oxygenated blood will then be distributed throughout the body. The left ventricle will pump oxygenated blood out through the **aorta** (largest artery in the body) that will be distributed to all organs and tissue of the body.

The right and left sides of the heart are separated by the septum. When the ventricles are pumping, the atria are relaxing, and vice versa. [10]

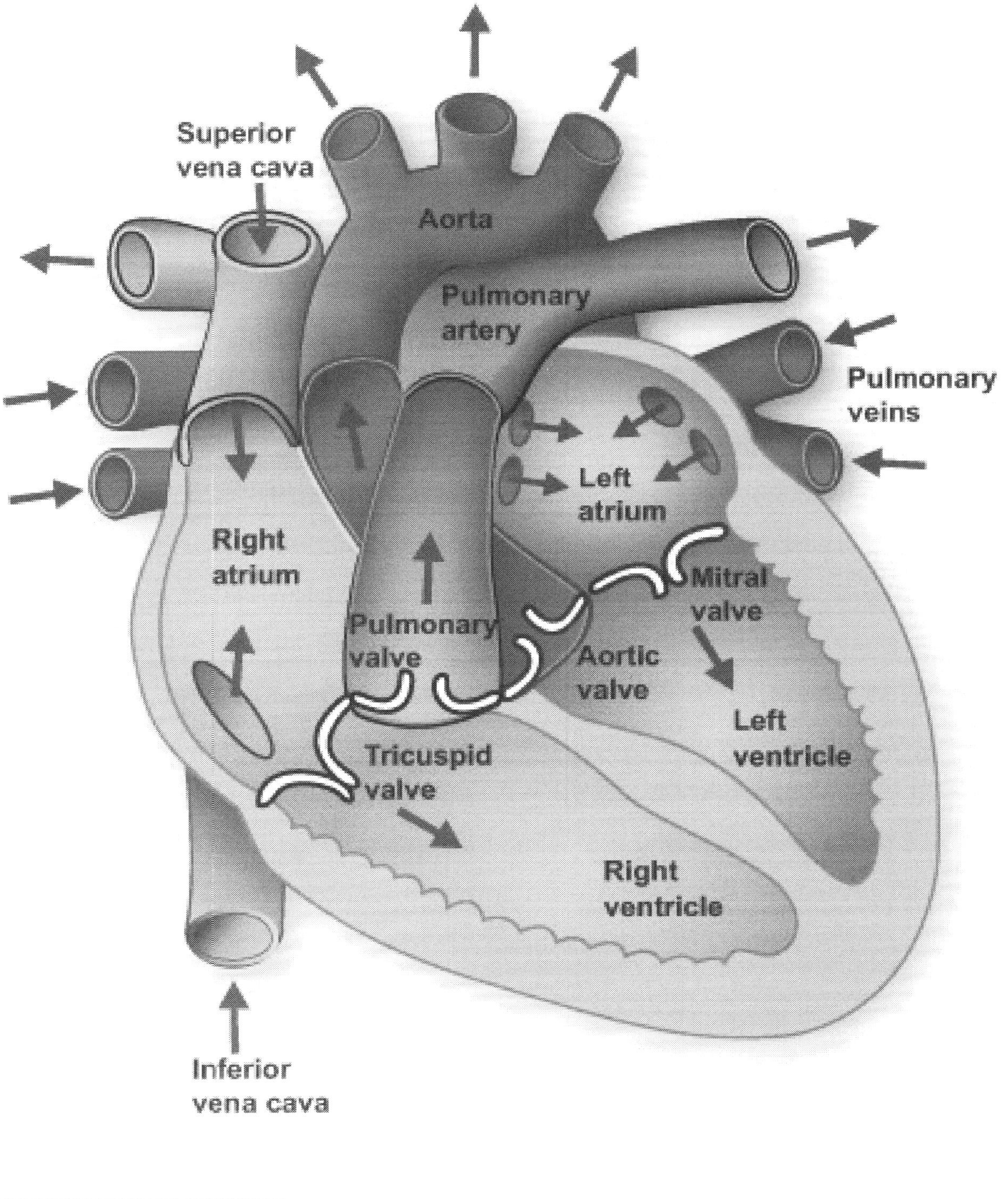

[10] Image taken from: http://www.texasheartinstitute.org/HIC/Anatomy/images/fig1_crosslg.jpg

The Cardiac Cycle

The **cardiac cycle** makes up the pumping action of the heart, and is the sequence of events which lead up to the contraction of the heart.

The contraction of the heart muscle (the myocardium) is called **systole.** When the heart muscle relaxes, it is called **diastole**. Remember the two numbers used in the measurement of blood pressure? The systolic, or top number, represents when the heart is contracting. The diastolic, or bottom number, represents the relaxing of the heart.

Stroke volume (SV) is the volume of blood being ejected from the left ventricle on every contraction. The stroke volume at rest is usually **70 ml**.

Heart rate (HR) is the number of times a heart beats per minute. When the body is at rest, heart rate can be about **72 beats per minute**.

Cardiac output (Q) is the amount of blood that is ejected from the left ventricle every minute. Heart rate and stroke volume produces cardiac output: **Q = HR * SV**

Cardiac output at rest is usually about **5 L per minute**.

HR (72 beats per minute) * SV (70 ml) = Q (5 L of blood per minute)

End-diastolic volume (EDV) is the amount of blood left in each ventricle after the heart muscle relaxes (diastole) during the cardiac cycle.

End-systolic volume (ESV) is the amount of blood left in each ventricle after the heart contracts. ESV at rest equals about 55 ml of blood.

Ejection fraction (EF) is the percentage of blood in the ventricle when the heart is in a relaxation (diastolic) state; but this blood actually gets pumped out during the contraction (systolic) phase.

The Frank-Starling Law states that the amount of blood left in each ventricle after the heart muscle relaxes (EDV) will significantly affect the SV; this is because a large amount of blood left in each ventricle after every contraction creates a greater stretch on the heart muscle. Over time, as the ventricle stretch increases, contractile force increases.. A normal EDV would be around 125 ml.

Effect of Exercise on Pulmonary and Cardiac Function

Pulmonary Function

Minute ventilation (VE) is the volume of air inhaled or exhaled in one minute. **At rest, minute ventilation is about 6 L/min**. Exercise increases **minute ventilation**, because breathing depth increases during physical activity.

Exercise also increases **respiratory rate**, evidenced by the increased number of breaths required as activity grows more intense. During maximal intensity exercise, minute ventilation may be 20 – 25 times higher than the typical 6 L/min that is seen at rest. This increase also causes **tidal volume** to increase.

Tidal volume is the amount of air entering or leaving the lungs in a single breath. The air that enters and leaves the lungs in a single breath is usually around **0.5 L to 4 L**.

Respiratory rate is the amount of breaths taken in one minute. Respiratory rate ranges from 12 breaths per minute to almost 50 breaths per minute, depending on exercise intensity.

In individuals who are healthy and who exercise regularly, exercise capacity is not limited by ventilation. Ventilatory capacity does not go under any changes with long term exercise in healthy individuals.

Cardiac Function
Two major modifications during exercise work to increase oxygen delivery to the working muscle tissue. They are shunting and vasodilation.

1. **Shunting** is a term used when blood is shunted away from all the vital (visceral) organs of the body to the exercising muscles. As exercise increases, **vasoconstriction** (narrowing of the blood vessels) takes place in the arterioles within the visceral organs; at the same time, **vasodilation** (widening of the blood vessels) takes place in the blood vessels (arterioles) in the muscle. This shunting causes a higher blood – and therefore **increased oxygen** – delivery to the working muscles, as well as less blood and oxygen from the visceral organs.

2. As aerobic exercise increases, so too will the vasodilation of the blood vessels in the working muscle. **Vasodilation** causes the total peripheral resistance (resistance of blood vessels to the flow of blood) to decrease. This accommodates the rise in cardiac output that occurs during exercise.

The Skeletal System

The skeletal system is composed of all the bones of the body, and can be divided into the **axial skeleton** and the **appendicular skeleton**.

The skeletal system provides support to the body; protection to all the internal organs of the body; and movement to the muscles that are attached to the bones by tendons.

Axial Skeleton
This skeleton includes all of the bones of the skull, vertebral column, ribs, and sternum. It supports and protects all of the internal organs.

Spine
The spine, or the vertebral column, provides the support of the skeletal structure. The human spine contains 33 vertebrae: seven cervical, twelve thoracic, five lumbar, five sacral, and four coccygeal (these bones are fused together to form one bone: the coccyx) vertebrae. Between each vertebra are intervertebral disks. These disks are flat and round, and are composed of fibrocartilaginous tissue.

Fibrocartilaginous Tissue
This tissue is strong and tough, but it allows for slight movement. Fibrocartilaginous tissue is composed of the annulus fibrosus which is the outer portion of the disk. The nucleus pulposus is a jelly-like substance in the middle of each disk that allows the vertebrae to absorb shock and bear weight.

A commonly-found abnormal curvature of the spine is **scoliosis**, a lateral or sideways deviation of the spine. It is an abnormal curve of the spine in the frontal plane.

Kyphosis is an excessive outward curvature of the spine that causes a hunching of the back. These curves occur in the **thoracic and sacral regions**, and develop in the fetus.

Lordosis curvature, on the other hand, is an inward curvature of the spine. These curves occur in the **cervical and lumbar** regions, developing after birth.

The human body has 24 ribs: twelve ribs on each side of the spine. There are 7 pairs of true ribs that attach to the sternum and spine, and 5 pairs of ribs do not attach to the sternum. The 8th, 9th, and 10th pair of ribs are connected to the ribs above them, and the 11th and 12th pair of ribs are called **floating ribs** (because their ends do not attach to anything).

The **sternum**, also called the breast bone, lies in the middle of the chest. It has three parts: the manubrium (superior), the body (middle), and the xiphoid process (inferior). The connection between the sternum and the ribs forms the ribcage, which serves as protection for the heart and lungs.

The Appendicular Skeleton
The other skeleton, the appendicular, consists of all the bones making up the arms, legs, pelvis, and pelvic girdle. This skeletal structure provides both movement and support.

The scapula and clavicles attach the limbs to the trunk of the body. The bones in the arms include the humerus, ulna, and radial bones. The glenoid fossa of the scapula attaches to the humerus, which in turn attaches to the ulna and radial bones that make up the forearm.

The pelvic and pelvis girdles provide attachment for the axial and appendicular skeleton together. The pelvic girdle consists of the hip bones (ilium, ischium, and pubis), the sacrum, and the coccyx. The femur (the largest bone in the body), the tibia, and the fibula form the leg.

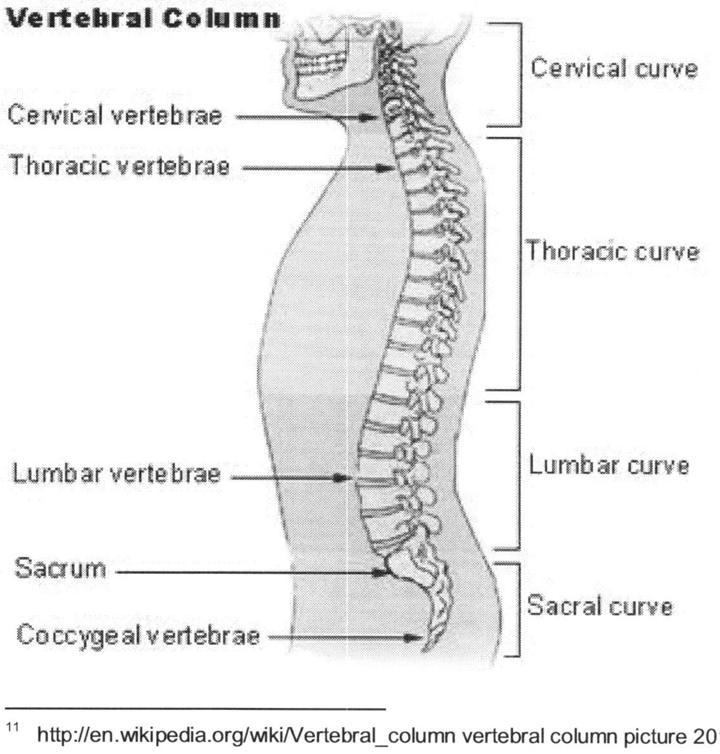

The bones of the spinal column are in specific order from the top of the spine to the end.

At the top of the spinal column are 7 cervical vertebra, then 12 thoracic vertebra, then 5 lumbar, five sacral, and four coccygeal (these bones are fused together to form one bone the coccyx) vertebrae.

On way to remember how many true vertebra bones are in the spinal column is to correlate their numbers with typical meal times:

We eat breakfast at 7:00 am. (7 cervical)

We eat lunch at 12:00 noon. (12 thoracic)

We eat dinner at 5:00 pm. (5 lumbar) [11]

[11] http://en.wikipedia.org/wiki/Vertebral_column vertebral column picture 2012

Muscles

There are three types of muscles:

1. Skeletal.

2. Cardiac.

3. Smooth. (Found in many parts of the body, including the blood vessels, the gastrointestinal tract, the bladder, and the uterus.)

Muscle Tissues
There are three different types of muscle tissue.

1. **Skeletal Muscle** is the most abundant tissue found in the human body, which accounts for 50% of the body's mass. Skeletal muscle's prime job is to provide contraction and relaxation to the muscle for movement, whether someone is getting out of bed, or bench pressing 150lbs. When you think of skeletal muscle think of the body's skeletal structure and these are the muscles that attach to it.

2. **Striated muscle** is also another term for skeletal muscle because of the striations you can see if looking at this muscle under a microscope that are made from the long and thin multinucleated fibers that are crossed with a regular pattern of fine red and white lines.

3. **Tendons** are what attach skeletal muscle to bones. If you think of bones as levers, the skeletal muscle is attached to the bones by tendons which give the body the ability for movement and mobility.

Skeletal Muscle
Skeletal Muscle is made up of many cells, called myofibers or myocytes. These cells are constructed and arranged to give the muscle its function. Skeletal muscle is orchestrated in a very fine fashion, consisting of the tendon attaching the muscle to the bone, all the way down to the myofibers.

The muscle is covered by a connective tissue called the **epimysium** which surrounds the entire muscle. Each muscle contains a bundle or fascicle that is surrounded by a layer of tissue called the **perimysium**; within each fascicle are about 150 myofibers lying parallel to each other, which are covered by a layer of connective tissue called the **endomysium**.

Within each myofiber is a structured system of organelles (the tiny "organs" of each cell) that make up the foundation for the muscle to work. And within each myofiber are multiple threads of myofibrils that contain **actin** and **myosin** filaments.

Almost all cells of the body have one nucleus (the control center of every cell), but myofibers contain more than one. Within each myofiber is the sarcoplasmic reticulum, which stores calcium until it is needed for muscle contraction.

Every cell has a plasma membrane; it surrounds a cell and separates the cell from its external environment. The myofiber's plasma membrane is called the **sarcolemma.**

Within the sarcolemma are many sodium voltage-gated channels that allow the muscle cell to be excited by action potentials. The sarcolemma also contain transverse tubules (T tubules), narrow tubes that are continuous with the sarcolemma. They form passageways that allow electrical impulses conducted by the sarcolemma to travel along the T tubules. These electrical impulses or action potentials are the trigger for muscle contraction.

Sarcomeres are segments of skeletal muscle; they are composed of actin and myosin filaments. The actin and myosin filaments are anchored to the Z-disc on the sarcomere.

The following page shows an illustration of what we just discussed.

Draw it out! Try your hand at reproducing this and all the images found in this section – it will help you remember the information better. First, study the image, noting the different parts of the drawing and their names. Then, either trace or look off of the image to create a duplicate. *Then,* once you are feeling confident with the information, try to draw it from memory. [12]

---

[12] Image taken from: Tianjin Rego Physical Education: Background reading 5 (2012) Retrieved October 30, 2012, from http://regopestudies.wikispaces.com/Background+Reading+5. All rights reserved.

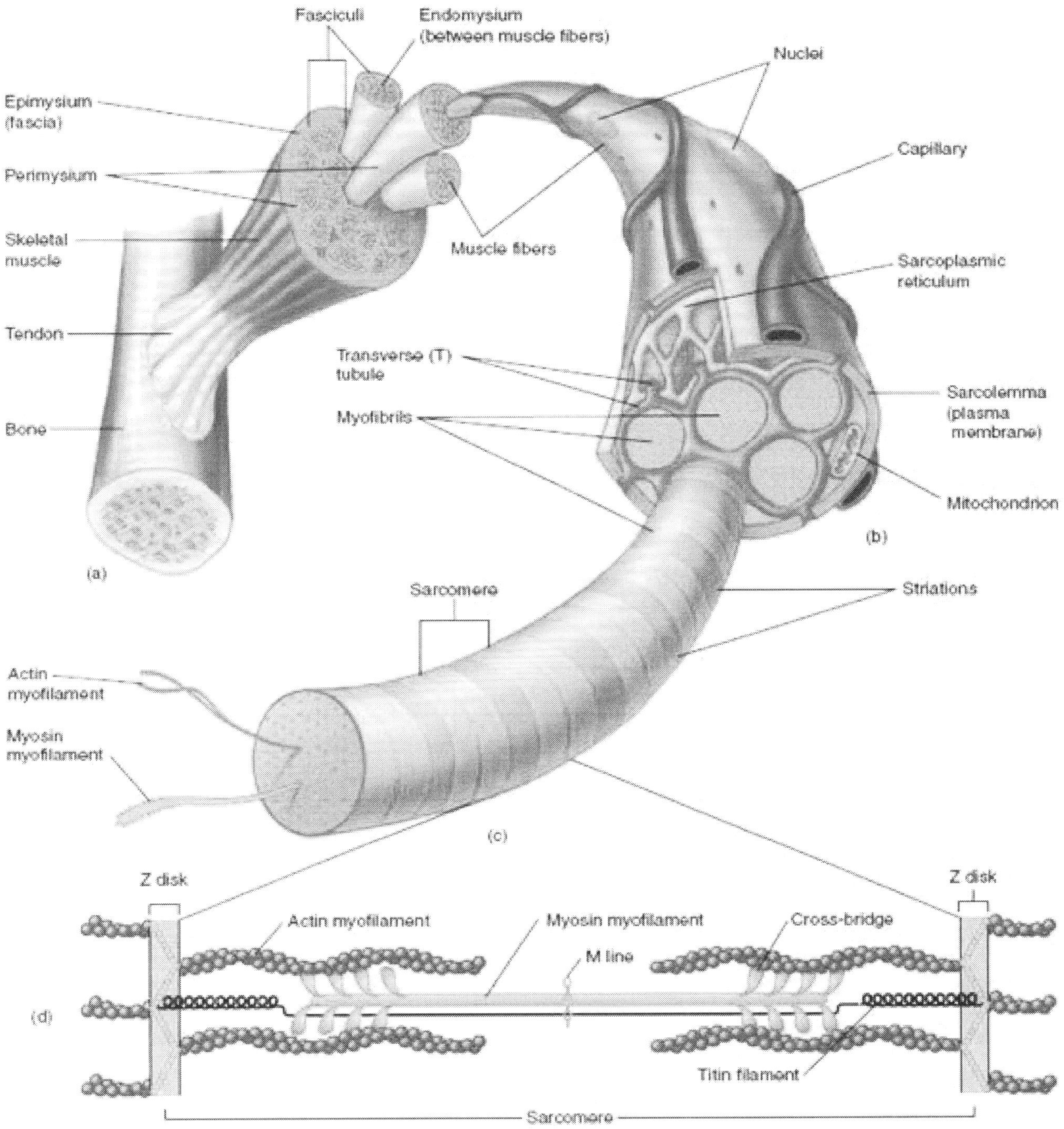
Fasciculi
Endomysium
(between muscle fibers)
Nuclei
Epimysium
(fascia)
Perimysium
Capillary
Skeletal
muscle
Muscle fibers
Sarcoplasmic
reticulum
Tendon
Transverse (T)
tubule
Myofibrils
Sarcolemma
(plasma
membrane)
Bone
Mitochondrion
(b)
(a)
Sarcomere
Striations
Actin
myofilament
Myosin
myofilament
(c)
Z disk
Z disk
Actin myofilament
Myosin myofilament
Cross-bridge
M line
(d)
Titin filament
Sarcomere

The two types of proteins which we just mentioned are:

1. Myosin: a large protein usually called the thick filament.
2. Actin: a smaller protein usually called the thin filament.

These proteins are organized into thin and thick **filaments** (long chains of subunit proteins) which repeat along the length of the myofibril in sections called sarcomeres. Myofilament is the term for the chains of (primarily) actin and myosin that pack a muscle fiber. These are the force-generating structures. Muscles contract by sliding the thin (actin) and thick (myosin) filaments along each other.

Sliding Filament Theory

Understanding the basics of how muscles are structured and how they work can aid in developing safe and effective strength programs for clients.

The sliding filament theory is the process by which muscles are believed to contract, relax, and/or produce force. Each muscle fiber consists of smaller fibers known as myofibrils. Myofibrils contain even smaller structures known as actin (thin) proteins and myosin (thick) filaments. When the filaments slide in and out, the muscle contracts.

There is a correlation between the length of a muscle and how much tension that muscle can generate. This is known as the **length-tension relationship**. A muscle can generate the greatest tension at its resting length. When tension is placed upon the muscle, that muscle will contract or lengthen (depending on the exercise).

How much the muscle is contracted or lengthened depends on the force that the muscle is able to generate. If a muscle is lengthened in excess, then it will not be able to produce enough force.

During an exercise, a repetition is made up of three distinct phases:

- Concentric phase (typically when you are lifting the weight).
- Transition or peak contraction phase (mid-point).
- Eccentric phase (typically when you are lowering the weight).

Remember the two phases of muscle movement, concentric and eccentric? The muscle shortens during the **concentric** part, and lengthens during the **eccentric** part.

> For example: During a squat exercise, the time when the body descends into the squat is considered the eccentric phase. The concentric phase occurs when the body ascends from a squat. During the concentric phase of a squat, when the body is ascending, the gluteus maximus shortens and acts as the prime mover.

The mechanism that allows the muscle to contract and relax is called **cross-bridge cycling.** Cross-bridge cycling is the production of movement and the generation of force by muscle cells.

Skeletal Muscle and the CNS

The **CNS** (the central nervous system) consists of the brain and spinal cord. The brain and spinal cord serve as the main processing centers for the entire nervous system; they control all the actions and movements of the body.

Action potentials – calls for specific functions – are sent from the CNS to stimulate the whole muscle for movement; the muscle fibers are then activated by a motor unit. Muscle fibers contract at the command of a motor nerve or motor unit. A **motor unit** is defined as a motor nerve and all the specific muscle fibers it innervates or activates.

When the muscle fibers' T-tubules are excited by an action potential, the inner portion of the muscle fiber is depolarized and muscle contraction starts to take place. The calcium that is stored inside the sarcoplasmic reticulum is released into the cell's **cytosol**, the liquid portion of the cell that is outside the nucleus.

Calcium is like a messenger. Once calcium is inside the cytosol, it looks for troponin and binds to it. When calcium is bonded to the regulatory filament troponin it causes the other regulatory filament, tropomyosin, to change shape.

The regulatory filaments troponin and tropomyosin are part of the thin filament actin. When tropomyosin is changing shape, active sites on actin are exposed. Myosin contains cross-bridge heads; when the active sites on actin are exposed, these cross-bridge heads will bind to them.

To contract a muscle, ATP causes a power stroke within the cross-bridge. That power stroke occurs as actin is pulled inward toward the center of the sarcomere. Actin and myosin are pulled towards each other, causing the sliding action. The muscle fiber will then shorten and generate force, causing muscle contraction.

Muscles stay contracted as long as calcium stays within the cytosol. Once calcium is pumped back into the sarcoplasmic reticulum from the calcium pump, myosin cross-bridge heads are broken from the active sites on actin. Tropomyosin will then cover these binding sites, and muscle relaxation can take place.

Cardiac Muscle

The difference between skeletal and cardiac muscle lies within their names. Skeletal muscle is attached to the skeletal structure and allows for the body's movement. Skeletal muscle is striated and is **voluntary** muscle.

Cardiac muscle, on the other hand, is the muscle that makes up the heart. Cardiac muscle is **involuntary**, which means self-contracting. Cardiac muscle is striated just like skeletal muscle.

Muscle Fibers

There are three types of muscle fibers in the human body: **Type I fibers, Type IIB, and Type IIA fibers**; each type of fiber serves a purpose, from holding our head up to sprinting around a track.

1. **Type I fibers** are **slow twitch fibers**; these fibers are most resistant to fatigue. They produce large amounts of ATP through the oxidative system. Type I fibers are developed through training and genetics. They are found in postural muscles, such as the neck and spine; they are also found in large amounts in marathon runners.

2. **Type IIB fibers** are **fast twitch fibers**; these fibers can produce bursts of power, but they fatigue quickly. ATP produced in the nonoxidative system is broken down rapidly in these fibers. These fibers are found in large amounts in sprinters.

3. **Type IIA fibers** are a combination of Type I and Type II fibers. ATP is produced in both the aerobic and anaerobic systems; Type IIA fibers can produce fast and strong muscle contractions. Even though these fibers are a combination of both Type I and Type II, they are still more prone to fatigue than Type I. Resistance training can turn Type IIB fibers into Type IIA fibers.

Muscle Classifications
Each muscle produces an action by attaching to a proximal and distal end of a bone. For every joint to be movable, there have to be two opposing muscle groups: an agonist and an antagonist.

An **agonist** is a prime mover that moves part of the body in one direction. **Antagonists** are the prime movers that move that body part it in the opposite direction. Muscles never work alone; when the agonist muscle is contracting the antagonist to that muscle is relaxing.

For example: When elbow flexion is taking place, the bicep (the agonist) will be contracting while the triceps will be relaxing (the antagonists). When elbow extension is taking place, the triceps (the antagonists) will be contracting and the bicep (the agonist) will be relaxing.

Concentric contractions are when the muscle shortens when contracting. (Example: The upward phase of a bicep curl.)

Eccentric contractions are when the muscle lengthens when contracting. (Example: The downward phase of a bicep curl.)

Isometric contractions occur when the muscle is neither shortening nor lengthening. (Example: Curling a dumbbell half way up and holding it in fixed position.)

Body Planes and Axes[13]

There are three body planes, referred to as the cardinal planes:

1. **Sagittal Plane**: This vertical plane divides the body into left and right sides.

2. **Transverse**: This horizontal plane divides the body into upper (superior) and lower (inferior) portions.

3. **Frontal (Coronal)**: This vertical plane divides the body into front (anterior) and back (posterior) portions.

These planes allow for human movement around an axis. An **axis** is a straight line around which an object rotates. Movement at the joint takes place in a plane about an axis. There are three axes of rotation.

1. **Mediolateral axis** lies perpendicular to the sagittal plane.

2. **Anteroposterior axis** lies perpendicular to the frontal plane.

3. **Longitudinal axis** lies perpendicular to the transverse plane.

[13] Image from: **http://wikidoc.org/images/3/34/BodyPlanes.jpg**

Movements and Examples
The **sagittal plane** allows flexion and extension movement. It rotates around the mediolateral axis. Some examples of this kind of movement would be walking or squatting.

The **frontal plane** allows for abduction/adduction, side flexion, and inversion/eversion. It rotates around the anteroposterior axis. Side bending and lateral arm lefts are examples of this kind of movement.

The **transverse plane** allows internal and external rotation, horizontal flexion and extension, and supination and pronation. It rotates around the longitudinal axis. This movement allows for activities such as throwing a baseball or performing a golf swing.

Anatomical Position
The body is standing erect and facing forward, with the arms at the sides and palms facing forward. The legs are parallel, and the toes are pointed forward.

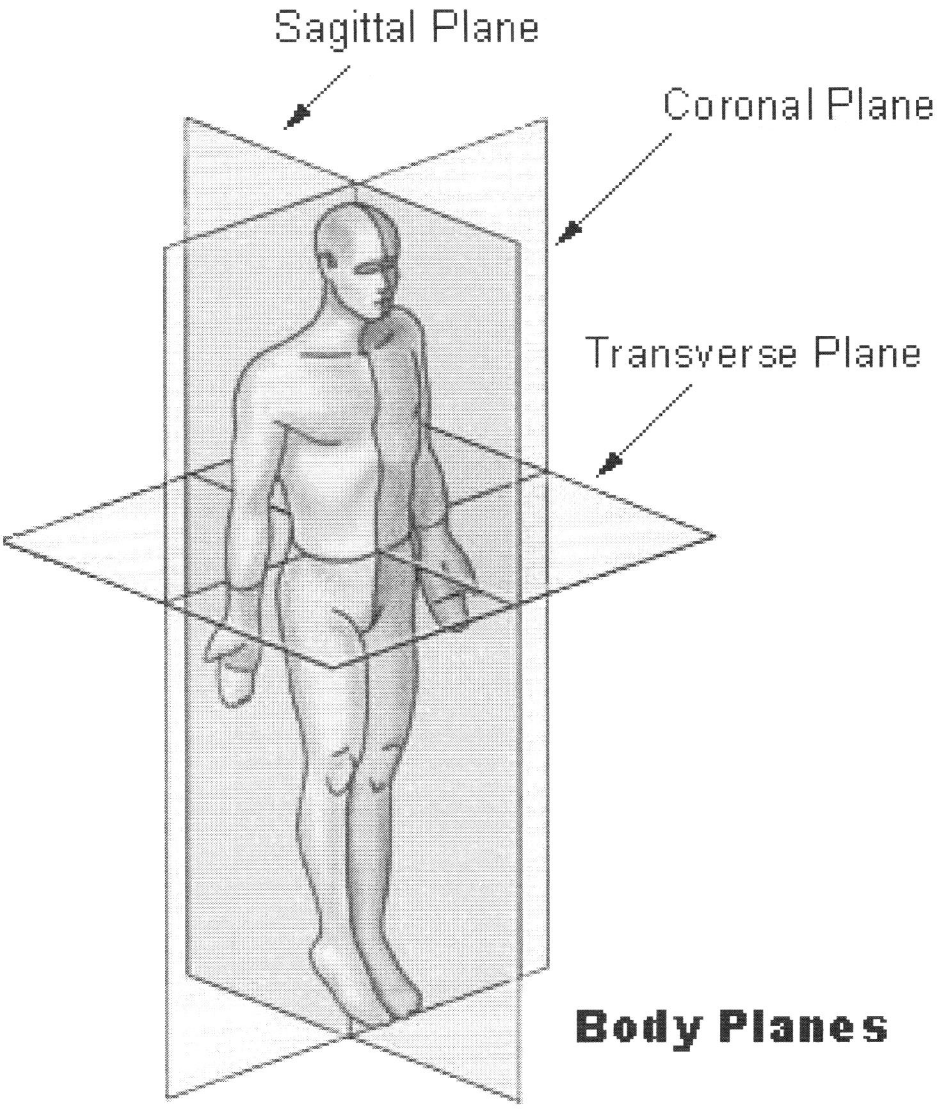

Anatomical Directions

Proximal: Nearest to the body center.

Distal: Away from the body center.

Superior (cranial): Towards the head.

Inferior (caudal): Towards the feet.

Anterior (ventral): Towards the front.

Posterior (dorsal): Towards the back.

Medial: Closer to the midline.

Lateral: Away from the midline.

Joints[14]

Joints are where two bones meet. The joints hold the bones together and allow mobility within the skeletal structure. Joints have three classifications:

1. **Fixed Joints (fibrous joints)**: Joints that have no movement. They are held together with fibrous (high strength) connective tissue. You will find these joints in the sutures of the skull. These immovable joints are also classified as **synarthrosis**.

2. **Slightly Movable Joints (cartilaginous joints)**: Joints found in the vertebrae of the spine and the ribcage. The vertebrae are connected to each other by cartilage pads which allows for slight movement. These slightly movable joints are also classified as **amphiarthrosis.**

3. **Freely Movable Joints (synovial joints)**: The most common joints found in the body. These joints allow the head to move from side to side, the knee and elbow to bend, and the shoulder to rotate. Freely movable joints are also classified as **diarthrosis.**

There are six different types of synovial joints in the human body.

Ball and socket joints allow circumduction, rotation, and angular movements in all planes (shoulder and hip).

Hinge joints allow the movements of flexion and extension in one plane (Knee and elbow).

Pivot joints allow for rotation around a central axis. This allows range of motion of the head and stability of the neck.

Saddle joints allow movement of flexion, extension, abduction, adduction, and circumduction and opposition. (Example: The thumb.)

---

[14] http://upload.wikimedia.org/wikipedia/commons/thumb/1/19/Joint.png/400px-Joint.png

Gliding joints allow for inversion and eversion. (Example: the ankle.)

Condyloid joints allow for circumduction, abduction, adduction, flexion, and extension. (Example: the wrist.)

Synovial joints contain articular cartilage, ligaments, synovial cavity, bursa, and joint capsules. All of these aspects allow the bones different ranges of motion.

When two bones conjoin together to form a synovial joint, the end surfaces of the bones are covered in articular cartilage. **Articular cartilage** is smooth and healthy tissue that allows joints to move easier; this allows bones to glide over each other with less friction.

Ligaments are the connective tissues which hold bones together. They can be found on the outside or inside of the joint cavity.

The joint capsule is a fibrous connective tissue that seals the joint space like an envelope. The joint capsule provides stability to the joint and surrounds the synovial cavity.

Synovial fluid is a lubricant inside the joint capsule. It is concealed by the synovial membrane. Synovial fluid's job is to cushion joints and make it easier for bones and cartilage to move past each other.

The Bursa is a sac filled with fluid that minimizes friction absorbs shock.

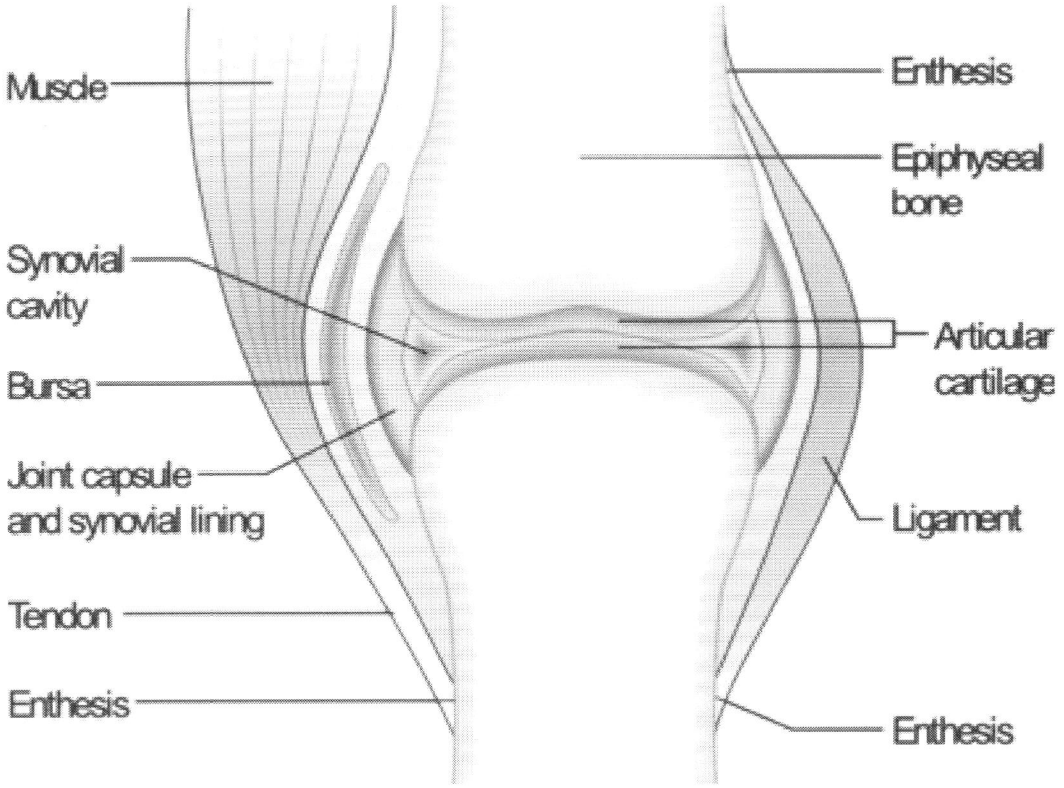

Movements Around a Joint

There are many terms that explain movements around a joint. These terms are:

1. **Flexion**: Movement that decreases the joint angle.

2. **Extension:** Movement that increases the joint angle.

3. **Adduction**: Movement toward the midline of the body.

4. **Abduction**: Movement away from the midline of the body.

5. **Rotation**: Movement either toward the midline or away from the midline of the body.

6. **Circumduction**: A combination of flexion, extension, abduction, and adduction movements.

7. **Supination**: Rotational movement at the radioulnar joint in the wrist. (Rotating the palm face up.)

8. **Pronation**: Rotational movement at the radioulnar joint in the wrist. (Rotating the palm face down.)

9. **Inversion**: Turning the sole of the foot toward the midline of the body.

10. **Eversion**: Turning the sole of the foot away from the midline of the body.

The following page shows a diagram of the above movements. Try them out yourself to get an idea of how they feel. [15]

[15] http://faculty.weber.edu/nokazaki/Human%20Anatomy/Notes/Articulations_files/image037.png

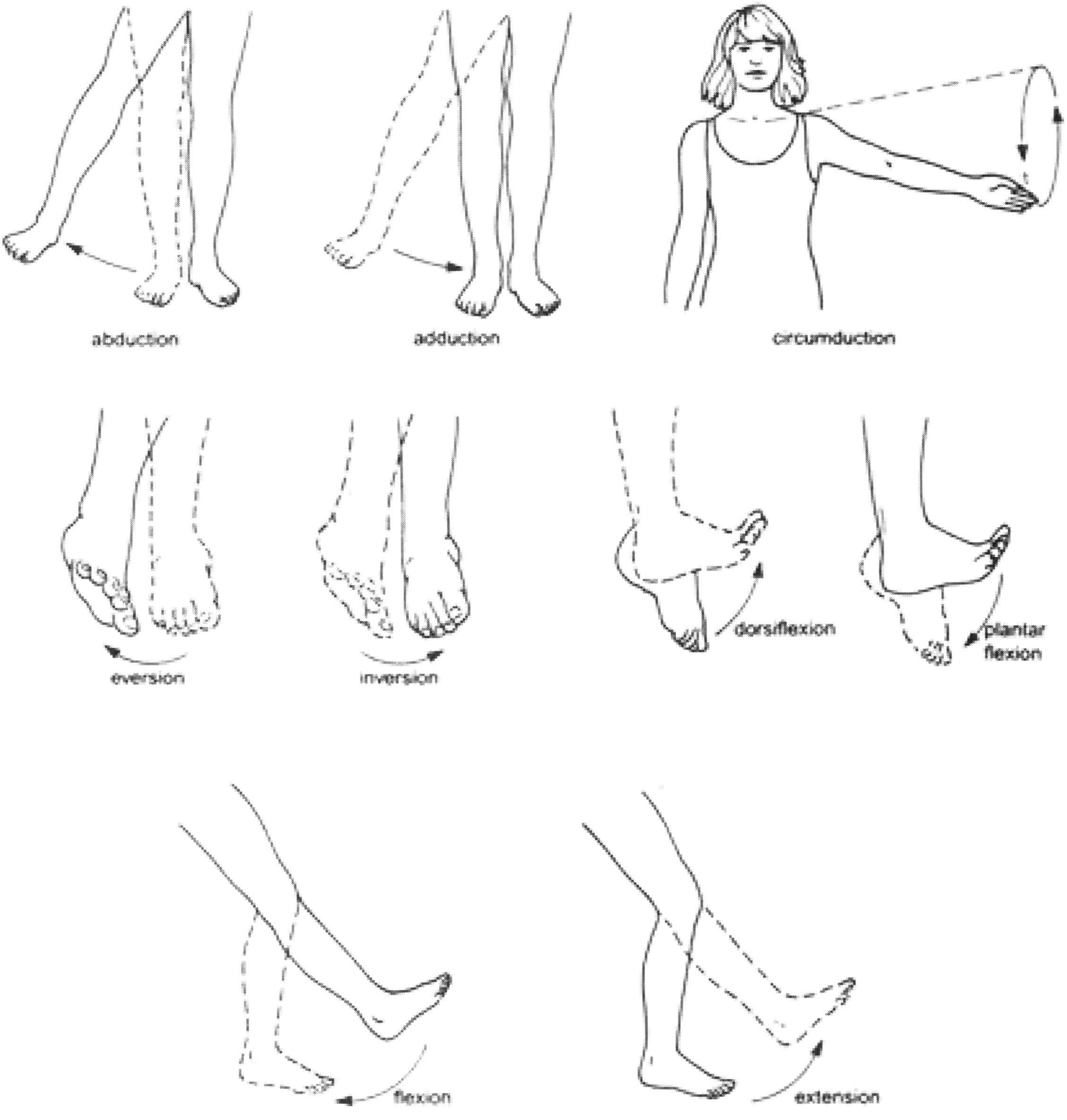
abduction
adduction
circumduction
eversion
inversion
dorsiflexion
plantar flexion
flexion
extension

Test Your Knowledge: Exercise Physiology and Related Exercise Science

1. What is another name for the bicuspid valve?

2. True/False: Valves prevent blood from flowing back into the ventricles.

3. Trace the route of blood through the heart

4. True/False: The diaphragm muscle is a respiratory muscle.

5. This movement increases the joint's angle and occurs in the sagittal plane around a mediolateral axis.

a) Rotation.
b) Flexion.
c) Circumduction.
d) Extension.

6. Which of the following is considered a saddle joint?

a) Hip.
b) Thumb.
c) Elbow.
d) Wrist.

7. Where does gas exchange take place inside the lungs?

a) Bronchioles.
b) Pharynx.
c) Trachea.
d) Alveoli.

8. Which bioenergetic pathway is sometimes called the "aerobic" pathway?

a) Oxidative.
b) Nonoxidative.
c) Anaerobic.
d) Phosphagen.

9. What explains how the muscles contract, relax, and/or produce force?

a) Myosin.
b) Sliding filament theory.
c) Sarcomeres.
d) Actin.

10. Which large protein, usually called the thick filament, is involved with muscle contraction?

a) Actin.
b) Sarcomere.
c) Myosin.
d) Nuclei.

11. During short duration and high intensity exercises, such as sprinting, which type of muscle fibers are primarily recruited?

a) Type IIB.
b) Type I.
c) Type IIA.
d) Type III.

12. What is the difference between type I and type II muscle fibers?

13. What is another name for the windpipe?

a) Larynx.
b) Trachea.
c) Pharynx.
d) Bronchioles.

14. What is the respiratory muscle that allows the human body to breath?

a) Femoris.
b) Triceps.
c) Diaphragm.
d) Pectoralis.

15. What term refers to the volume of blood that is ejected out of every ventricle per contraction?

a) Cardiac Output.
b) Stroke Volume.
c) Heart Rate.
d) End-systolic volume.

16. True/False: During maximal intensity exercise, minute ventilation may be 20-to-25 times higher than the typical 6 L/min that is observed under resting conditions.

17. What is the term used to describe the amount of blood ejected every minute from the left ventricle?

a) Heart rate,
b) Stroke volume.
c) Ejection Fraction.
d) Cardiac Output.

18. What is the term used for when blood is being pulled away from all the vital (visceral) organs of the body to the exercising muscles?

a) Vasodilation.
b) Shunting.
c) Vasoconstriction.
d) Systole.

19. Name a beneficial Cardiac Adaption from long-term cardiovascular exercise?

a) Decreases resting heart rate.
b) Slight decrease in resting blood pressure.
c) Increase in stroke volume.
d) All of the above.

20. True/False: The Appendicular skeleton includes the bones of the skull, vertebral column, ribs, and sternum.

21. Intervertebral disks are composed of ______ tissue.

a) Epithelial.
b) Fibrocartilaginous.
c) Muscle.
d) Heart.

22. What curvature causes a hunching of the back due to excessive outward curving of the spinal column?

a) Kyphosis.
b) Scoliosis.
c) Lordosis.
d) Hyperlordosis.

23. When elbow flexion is taking place, the bicep will contract while the triceps relax. Which prime mover is the agonist?

24. What tissue holds bones together?

a) Tendon.
b) Joint capsule.
c) Articular cartilage.
d) Ligament.

Test Your Knowledge: Exercise Physiology and Related Exercise Science – Answers

1. The **Mitral valve** is another name for the bicuspid valve that separates the left atrium from the left ventricle.

2. **True**.

3. See chart on page 70.

4. **True**. The diaphragm is a respiratory muscle that is essential for humans to breath.

5. **d) Extension.**

6. **b) Thumb**. The saddle joint provides flexion, extension, abduction, adduction, and circumduction.

7. **d) Alveoli**. Alveoli are tiny air sacs where gases are exchanged between the lungs and blood.

8. **a) Oxidative**. The oxidative system is also called the aerobic pathway because oxygen is required for this pathway to work.

9. **b) Sliding filament theory**.

10. **c) Myosin**.

11. **a) Type IIB**. Type IIB fibers are fast twitch fibers; these fibers can produce bursts of power, but they fatigue quickly.

12. **Type II fibers** are for high intensity and short duration exercises (sprinting and weightlifting). **Type I fibers** are for low intensity and long duration exercise (marathon running).

13. **b) Trachea**.

14. **c) Diaphragm**.

15. **b) Stroke volume**.

16. **True**.

17. **d) Cardiac Output**.

18. **b) Shunting**.

19. **d) All of the above**.

20. **False**. The Appendicular Skeleton includes all of the bones that make up the arms, legs, pelvis, and pelvic girdle. This skeletal structure provides for movement and support. The axial skeleton includes the bones of the skull, vertebral column, ribs, and sternum. It provides the support and protection of all the internal organs.

21. b) Fibrocartilaginous. Between each vertebra are intervertebral disks. These disks are flat and round and are composed of fibrocartilaginous tissue. This tissue is strong and tough; it allows for slight movement.

22. a) Kyphosis. Kyphosis curvature is excessive outwards of the spinal that causes hunching of the back. These are curves in the thoracic and sacral regions.

23. Bicep.

24. d) Ligament.

Chapter 5: Nutrition and Weight Management

Health is not solely dependent upon how much people exercise their bodies; proper nutrition, or how one feeds and fuels the body, is essential to a healthy lifestyle. However, how can you tell if a person is healthy? A common misconception in our society today is that weight is an indicator of health. In reality, many factors influence individual health, and what is healthy for one person may not be healthy for another. Never use terms such as "skinny" or "fat." Those are unprofessional, and woefully inadequate, descriptors. Instead, start thinking in terms of body composition.

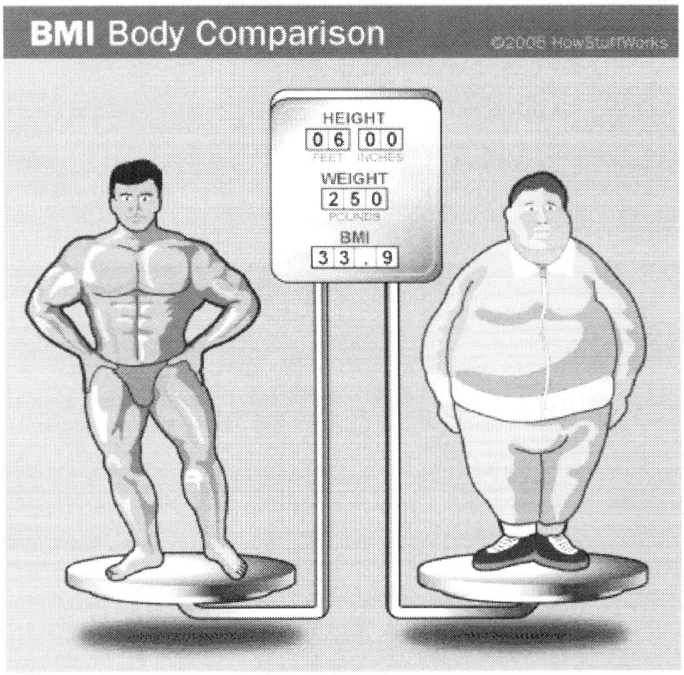

These individuals may weigh the same, but they are at very different levels of health![16]

Body Composition Assessment

Bodies are made up of varying amounts of water, proteins, minerals, and fat. Assessing body composition can determine the amount of fat, bone and muscle in an individual's body. In the human body, muscle tissue takes up less space than fat tissue, but weighs significantly more. Therefore, body composition and weight combined determine the leanness and fitness of an individual.

Why is it Necessary

Even though the amount of muscle and fat in a person's body determines how they look and feel, it is not enough just to know an individual's weight in order to make recommendations. People of equal height and body weight may have completely different levels of health, because they have different body

[16] Image from: http://srxa.files.wordpress.com/2012/07/bmi-comparison.gif

compositions. Assessing the amounts of body fat, type of fat, and amounts of muscle in a person's body explicitly explains how healthy they are, regardless of how they may look externally.

How to Assess

There are many different methods of assessing body composition. It has recently become known that standard Body Mass Index tables using an individual's age, height, and weight to determine their fat composition tend to incorrectly indicate that individuals are overweight. Some common practical methods include using calipers or skinfolds and conducting bioelectrical impedance analysis (BIA). Most methods of body fat composition measurement have a 3 – 4% rate of error, which means that if an individual is measured to have 20% body fat, they could actually have as low as 17% or as high as 23% body fat. This error percentage depends highly on correct measurement, and can fluctuate depending on the skill of the technician taking the measurements.

Skinfolds

This method involves measuring the subcutaneous fat thickness at specific sites of the body using a caliper. The individual's skin should be dry and free of oils and lotions. Measurements should not be taken immediately after exercise due to the shift of body fluid to the skin. [ii]

The steps below outline how to perform skinfold measurements:

1. Take all skinfold measurements on the right side of the body.
2. Carefully identify and mark the skinfold sites
3. Place the thumb and index finger approximately 3 inches (8 cm) perpendicular to the skinfold, following the natural cleavage lines of the skin
4. Grasp the skinfold firmly with the thumb and index finger just slightly less than 1/2 inch (1 cm) above the marked site to be measured
5. Do not release the skinfold during the measurement.
6. Place the jaws of the caliper approximately 1/2 inch (1 cm) below the thumb and index finger; always release the caliper jaw pressure slowly
7. The skinfold measurement should be taken 4 seconds after the pressure is released. Measure the skinfold to the nearest 1/2 to 1 mm.

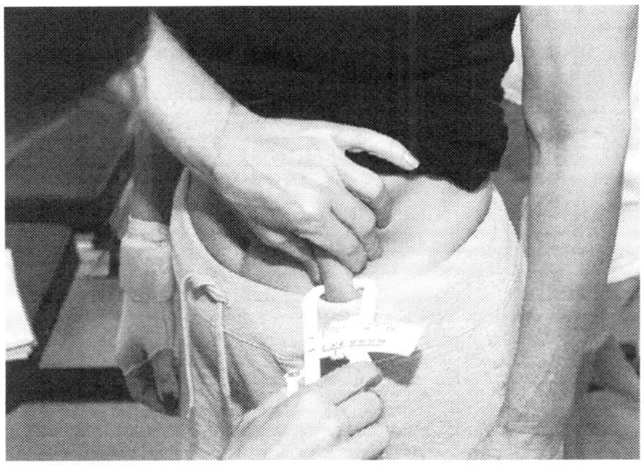 [17]

A woman being measured using the skinfold method.

[17] Image from: http://cathe.com/wp-content/uploads/2012/02/shutterstock_58153072.jpg

A minimum of two measurements should be taken at each site listed below, taken in a rotational order rather than by taking consecutive readings at the same site. If your values differ by more than 1 mm, take additional measurements.

Measuring Sites for Women:

Triceps: Take a vertical fold on the posterior midline of the upper arm halfway between the top of the shoulder and the elbow joint. Keep the elbow extended and relaxed.

Thigh: Take a vertical fold on the front aspect of the thigh, midway between the top of the knee cap and the hip.

Suprailium: Take a diagonal fold above the crest of the ilium (hip-bone), at the spot where an imaginary line comes down from the anterior line of the armpit (anterior axillary line).

Measuring Sites for Men:

Chest: Take a diagonal fold half the distance between the anterior axillary line (line of armpit) and nipple.

Abdomen: Take a vertical fold at a lateral distance approximately 2 cm (3/4 inch) to the right of the umbilicus (belly button).

Thigh: Take a vertical fold on the front aspect of the thigh, midway between the top of the knee cap and the hip.

See the following pages for illustrations.

Triceps

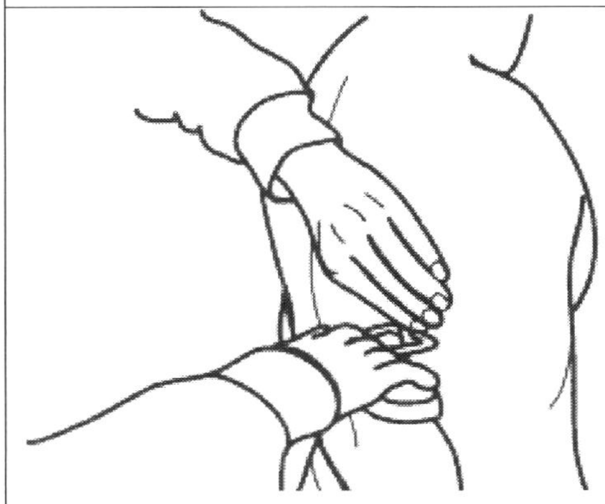

Arm held freely to the side of the body

- Vertical fold
- Posterior midline of the upper arm
- Halfway between the acromion (shoulder) and olecranon processes (elbow)

Chest

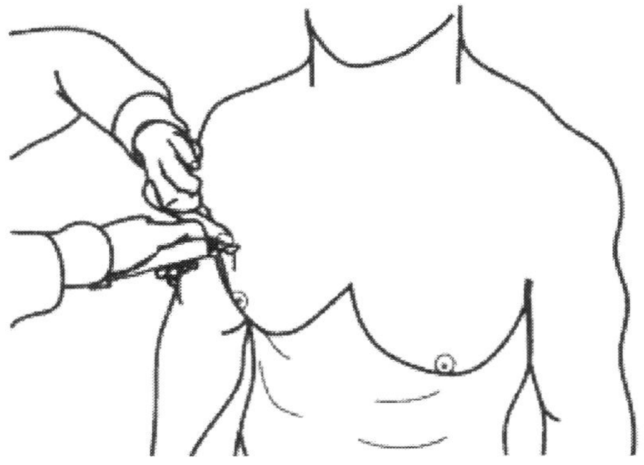

- Diagonal fold
- Men: one-half the distance between the anterior axillary line (crease of the underarm) and the nipple.
- Women: one-third of the distance between the anterior axillary line and the nipple

Mid-Axillary

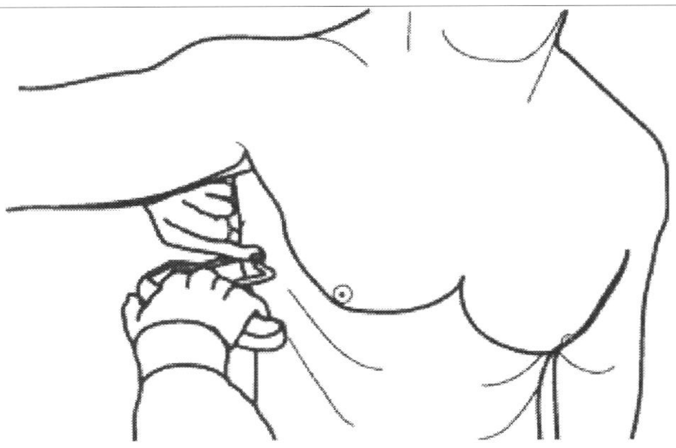

- Vertical or Horizontal fold
- Mid-axillary line at the level of the xiphoid process of the sternum

Subscapular

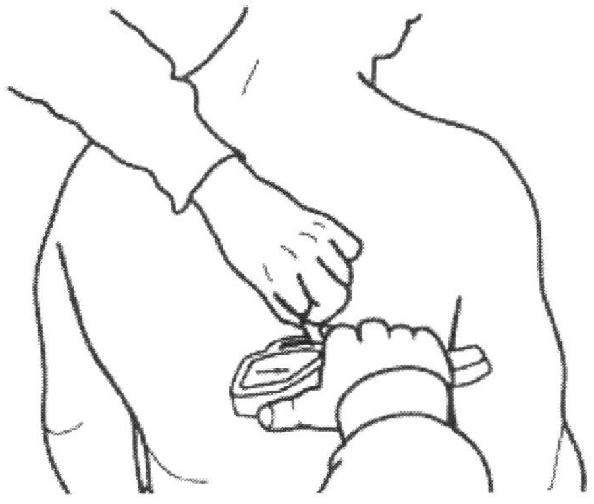

- Diagonal fold
- 1 to 2 cm below the inferior angle of the scapula

Suprailiac

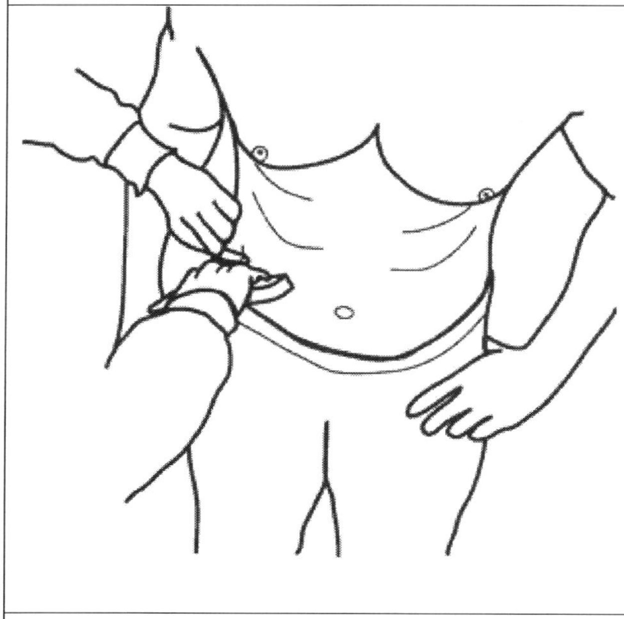

- Diagonal fold
- Anterior axillary line (modern technique)
  - Immediately superior to the iliac crest
  - In line with the natural angle of the iliac crest taken
- Mid-axillary line (traditional technique)
  - Superior to the iliac crest

Abdominal

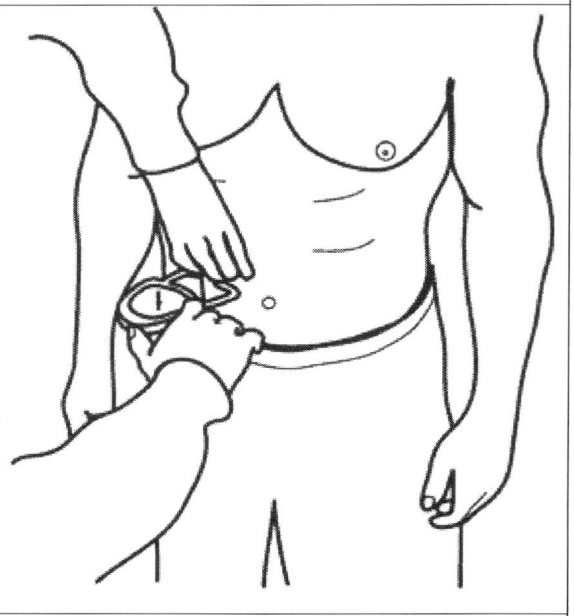

- Vertical (modern technique)
  - 2 cm or 1" to the right side of the umbilicus
- Horizontal fold (traditional)
  - 2 cm to the right side of the umbilicus

Thigh

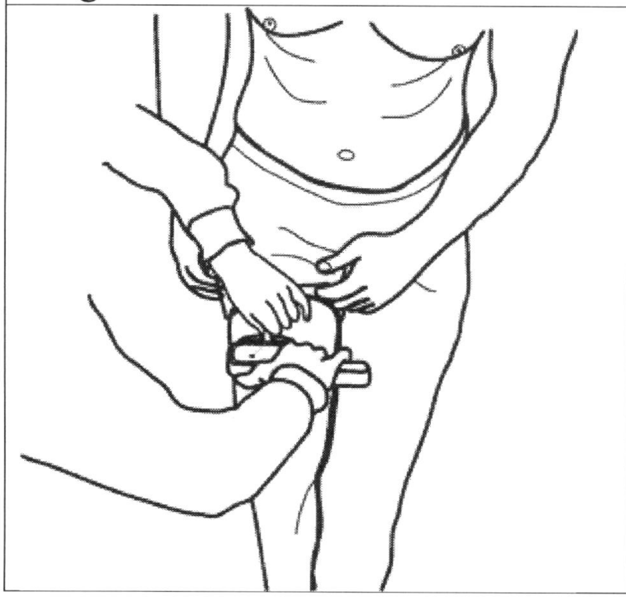

Other Sites

Biceps

- Vertical fold
- Anterior aspect of the arm over the belly of the biceps muscle
- 1 cm above the level used to mark the triceps site

Calf

- Vertical fold
- Maximum circumference of calf on the midline of medial border

Bioelectrical Impedance Analysis

The most prevalent component of the human body is water, which makes up approximately 55 – 78% of a human body. Bioelectrical Impedance Analysis (BIA) is based on the fact that this fluid is capable of electrical conduction. A safe, low-level current is administered and flows through these intracellular and extracellular fluids of the body in order to determine body composition, though patients cannot feel the current passes through their bodies.

[18]

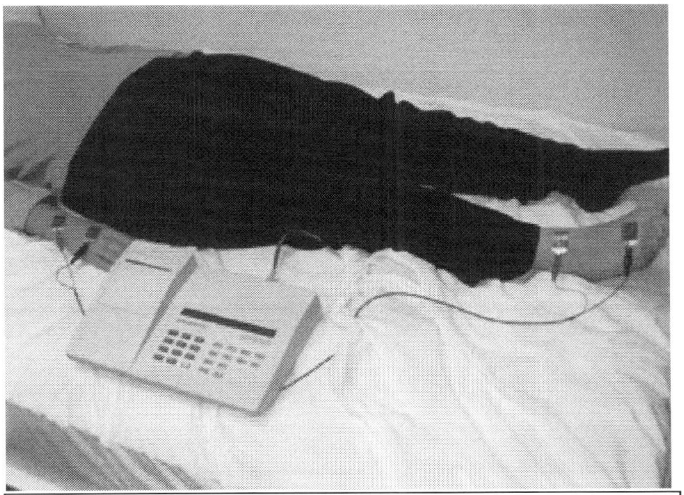

A woman having a BIA performed.

This BIA technique calculates an individual's total body water, from which fat free weight can be estimated. This test is administered while the patient lies on a testing table or floor and electrodes are attached to their hands and feet. This method of body composition analysis, although more lengthy and expensive, is believed to be more accurate than skinfold measurements.

Implications of Assessment

The minimum recommended level of total body fat for men is 5% and for women is 15%. The ranges for optimal health are 10 – 25% body fat for men and 18 – 30% body fat for women. These percentages and ranges tend to be lower for athletes in order to enhance body productivity and performance.

Understanding How Fat Distributions Relate to Disease

Excessive accumulation of fat at specific sites in the body is an important health risk factor. Stomach fat, in particular, is closely related to insulin resistance and diabetes within an individual. There are greater health risks if an individual carries excess weight around the abdomen (apple-shaped), as opposed to the hips and thighs (pear-shaped). Apple shape is also referred to as **anthroid**, as it is seen more-commonly in males; while the pear shape, seen more-commonly in females, is called **gynoid**.

[18] Image from: http://www.ohsu.edu/xd/research/centers-institutes/octri/resources/octri-research-services/images/BIA-for-website.JPG

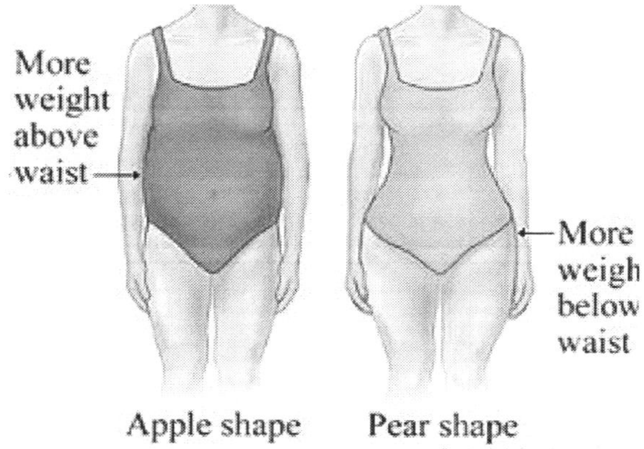

Waist-to-Hip Ratios for Men and Women[19]
A waist-to-hip ratio (WHR) is a fraction that represents the circumference of the waist divided by the circumference of the hip. The waist measurement is taken from the narrowest point, while the hips measurement is taken from the widest point (around the buttocks region. To obtain the ratio, divide the waist measurement by the hip measurement. This common physical measurement can be used to determine an individual's level of healthiness.

Ideal WHR Ranges
For women ages 18 – 59 the ideal WHR range is below .87, while for women 60 or older the ideal range is below .91. In women, the positive health effects of maintaining ideal waist-to-hip ratios are optimal levels of estrogen and lowered susceptibility to diabetes, cardiovascular disorders, and ovarian cancers. For men ages 18 – 59 the ideal WHR range is below .96, while for men 60 or older the ideal range is below 1.04. In men, the positive health effects are higher fertility and lower susceptibility to prostate and testicular cancers.

The World Health Organization outlines the protocol for measuring waist-to-hip ratios: [xi]

1. Measure the waist circumference at the end of several consecutive natural breaths, at a level parallel to the floor, midpoint between the top of the iliac crest and the lower margin of the last palpable rib in the mid axillary line.

2. Measure the hip circumference at a level parallel to the floor, at the largest circumference of the buttocks.

3. Make both measurements with a stretch-resistant tape that is wrapped snugly around the subject, but not to the point that the tape is constricting. Keep the tape level and parallel to the floor at the point of measurement.

4. Ensure that the subject is standing upright during the measurement, with arms relaxed at the side, feet evenly spread apart, and body weight evenly distributed.

[19] Image from: http://www.metrolic.com/wp-content/uploads/2011/03/apple.jpg

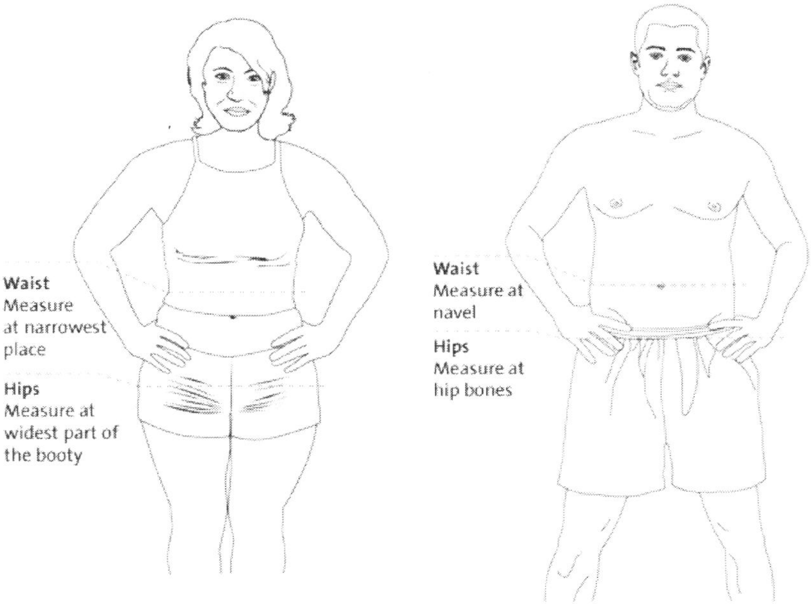

Waist-to-hip ratio measurements.[1]

Eating Disorders

In this weight-obsessed society, eating disorders are rampant and occur when an individual has an unhealthy relationship with their body or with food. When an individual becomes obsessed with food and weight to the point of unhealthy restrictions or practices, the results can include serious, sometimes life-threatening, physical complications.

Treatments for eating disorders must be designed with the highest level of effectiveness in mind for the individual, and usually involve psychotherapy, nutrition education, family counseling, medications, and hospitalization. The most common eating disorders are anorexia nervosa, bulimia nervosa, and binge-eating disorder. Below are descriptions of these common disorders according to multiple national eating disorder support groups.

Anorexia Nervosa is seen most commonly in young women in their late teens and early twenties, and is characterized by severe limitations to food intake, or the refusal to eat. According to the most current edition of the Diagnostic and Statistical Manual of Mental Disorders (DSM-IV) there are four criteria that must be present to achieve a diagnosis of Anorexia Nervosa:

- The person must refuse to maintain body weight over a minimal normal weight for age and height or have a failure to make expected weight gain during a defined period of growth, resulting in a body weight 15% lower than expected.
- Though underweight, the person experiences intense fear of gaining weight or becoming fat.
- The person must have a disturbance in the way his or her body weight, size, or shape is experienced and also experience undue influence of body weight, or shape on self-evaluation, or denial of the seriousness of the current body weight.
- Finally, (for women) amenorrhea must be present. Amenorrhea is the absence of at least three consecutive menstrual cycles when otherwise expected to occur.

Additionally, according to the Mayo Clinic, Anorexia Nervosa causes numerous complications like arrhythmias or a severe lack of essential nutrients, and can be fatal, even when someone is not severely underweight. If a person becomes severely malnourished, every organ in the body can be damaged, including the brain, heart, and kidneys. Additionally, this damage may not be fully reversible, even once the disorder is under control. [iv]

The potential complications from anorexia nervosa include: [iv]

- Anemia, kidney problems, and/or death.
- Heart problems, such as mitral valve prolapse, abnormal heart rhythms and heart failure.
- Bone loss, increasing risk of fractures later in life.
- In females, absence of a period. In males, decreased testosterone.
- Gastrointestinal problems, such as constipation, bloating or nausea.
- Electrolyte abnormalities, such as low blood potassium, sodium and chloride.
- Mental health issues and disorders.

Bulimia Nervosa. As opposed to anorexia nervosa, which limits the amount of food consumed, bulimia nervosa is characterized by the cyclical bingeing and purging of foods. **Bingeing** occurs when an individual discretely consumes more food than most other people would eat in a similar occurrence over a period of time, typically while feeling a lack of control of said food consumption. According to the national support group, Bulimia Nervosa exists when:

- Bingeing and compensatory behaviors occur on average 2 times weekly or more for a period of at least 3 months.
- When the behaviors are not exclusively those of Anorexia Nervosa.
- When self-evaluation is unduly influenced by body shape or weight.

Individuals with bulimia are often very concerned about gaining weight and intensely fear getting fat. These individuals may engage in purging or non-purging behaviors, such as vomiting, using laxatives, using diuretics, using enemas, fasting, or exercising excessively, which are often conducted in secret because of the shame and disgust associated with the processes.[iii] Bulimia nervosa may cause numerous serious and even life-threatening complications. Possible complications include: [iv]

- Dehydration, which can lead to major medical problems, such as kidney failure.
- Heart problems, such as an irregular heartbeat (arrhythmia) and heart failure.
- Severe tooth decay and gum disease.
- Absence of a period in females.

- Digestive problems, and possibly a dependence on laxatives to have bowel movements.
- Anxiety and depression.
- Drug and alcohol abuse.

Binge-Eating Disorder. The bingeing which occurs in bulimia nervosa can also stand as its own disorder. Binge-Eating Disorder (BED). In BED, recurrent bingeing episodes (twice weekly or more, for a period of at least six months) are associated with at least three of the following characteristics: [iii]

- Eating until uncomfortable.
- Eating when not physically hungry.
- Eating rapidly.
- Eating alone for fear of being embarrassed by how much food is being consumed.
- Feeling disgusted, depressed or guilty after the episode of overeating.

The negative feelings associated with BED may in turn trigger more bingeing behavior. However, BED is not associated with inappropriate compensatory behaviors such as those found in Bulimia Nervosa or Anorexia Nervosa, so people with BED are often either overweight or obese due to the extra calories they ingest. [iii]

Complications that may be linked with binge-eating disorder include: [iv]

- Depression.
- Suicidal thoughts.
- Insomnia.
- Obesity.
- High blood pressure.
- Type 2 diabetes.
- High cholesterol.
- Gallbladder disease and other digestive problems.
- Heart disease.
- Some types of cancer.
- Joint pain.

- Muscle pain.
- Headache.
- Menstrual problems.

Health Risks which come with High and Low Body Fat
Many problems are associated with high body fat, such as obesity, chronic disease, absent menstrual periods, hypertension, elevated blood lipids (fats and cholesterol), diabetes mellitus, cardiovascular disease, respiratory dysfunction, gall bladder disease, some joint diseases, and even death.

On the other hand, health problems associated with low body fat include, but are not limited to, heart failure, organ shut down, absent menstrual periods, delay in growth, osteoporosis, constipation, edema, and even death.

Knowledge of "Fat"
In the human body, total body fat consists of essential fat and storage fat. Both are necessary for healthy body function. **Essential** fat, as the name suggests, is necessary for normal body function and occurs in the marrow of bones, in the heart, lungs, liver, spleen, kidneys, intestines, muscles, and lipid-rich tissues throughout the central nervous system. It should be noted that women have a higher essential fat percentage than men for the functions of childbirth and other hormonal functions.

On the other hand, **storage** fat accumulates in adipose tissue and is located around internal organs. Storage fat serves many functions, such as the protection of internal organs in the chest and abdomen, as well as insulation for the conservation of body heat.

Calories

In reality, a calorie is a unit of energy. It is the amount of energy required to raise the temperature of one gram of water by one degree Celsius. But dietary calories are actually kilocalories, in that they are the amount of energy required in order to raise the temperature of one **kilogram** of water by one degree Celsius. Dietary calories are the energy in food. The body constantly needs energy in order to complete normal day-to-day actions and uses the calories from food to keep functioning. [v]

Caloric Expenditure and Requirements for Exercise and Daily Activity
An individual's caloric intake depends on a number of variables including their current weight, height, and level of healthiness. On average, the "normal" person should intake no more than 2000 calories per day and should get moderate levels of exercise for **at least** 150 minutes per week (that is, 20 minutes per day or 30 minutes 5 times a week). [xii]

Amount of calories that equal one pound of body fat
Mathematically, 3,500 calories equals about 1 pound (0.45 kilogram) of fat. An individual would need to burn 3,500 calories more than they take in to lose 1 pound. So, if someone wanted to lose the recommended maximum of 2 pounds per week, they would have to eat a deficit of 1,000 calories every day to achieve their goal.

This can be mathematically calculated as: 1,000 * 7 = 7,000÷ 2 = 3,500 = 2 pounds.

Healthy Fats versus Non-Healthy Fats
As mentioned above, some types of fat are good for the body and essential to an individual's existence. Saturated fats and "trans" fats are bad, because they are complex fats, which are hard for the body to dissolve and break down.

These types of fats increase cholesterol levels and risk of developing chronic diseases. Mono-unsaturated fats and poly-unsaturated fats are good, because they lower cholesterol and, in fact, reduce the risk of acquiring certain diseases.

The amounts of good versus bad fats that a person eats, rather than the total amount of fat in the diet, is what matters most when it comes to cholesterol and health. Eating items labeled as low fat or fat-free does not ensure their health; and it certainly does not mean unlimited consumption without weight gain. Fat is not the only thing which contains calories – a food can be made entirely out of sugar, and contain 800 calories, while still remaining "fat-free."

Knowledge, balance, and moderation are the keys to a balanced and nutritious diet.

Nutrition

Basic Knowledge of the Food Pyramid
The food pyramid, now known as "My Plate" exists as a simple representation of the breakdown and amount of nutrients that an individual should consume every day. The next page shows a visual representation of the previously used "My Pyramid."

The USDA has now replaced the harder-to-read Food Pyramid with the simple MyPlate. [xii] This visual is easily able to help people keep track of how much to eat from each food group. The new easy-to-use website offers healthy recipes, healthy eating tips, and even personalized diet plans based on size, age, and activity level!

The new visual representation of "MyPlate" is shown below: [20]

[20] Image from: www.choosemyplate.gov

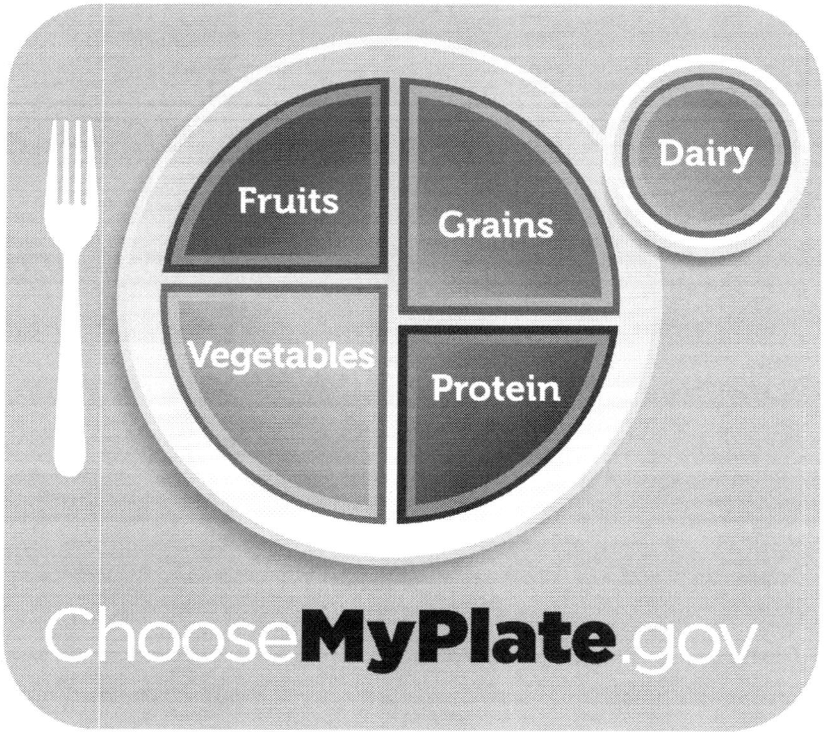
Fruits
Grains
Dairy
Vegetables
Protein
ChooseMyPlate.gov

Macronutrients
There are three major types of macronutrients: carbohydrates, lipids, and amino acids (proteins).

Carbohydrates
Carbohydrates are the most important source of energy for the body, which converts carbohydrates into glucose (blood sugar). This sugar is used for energy for cells, tissues, and organs, and any extra sugar is stored in the liver and muscles for when it is needed.[viii]

Carbohydrates can be considered simple or complex, depending on their structure. Simple carbohydrates include sugars found naturally in foods such as fruits, vegetables, milk, and milk products, as well as sugars added during food processing and refining. Complex carbohydrates include whole grain breads and cereals, starchy vegetables, and legumes. [viii]

Carbohydrates provide four calories per gram ingested. The recommended sources for carbohydrates include: "whole grains, vegetables, fruits, and beans. Other highly processed foods also contain carbohydrates; however an overabundance of processed foods such as white rice and bread, pastries, sugared sodas, etc. may contribute to weight gain while promoting heart disease and diabetes.

Lipids
Lipids are various substances which are not soluble in water. They are necessary for healthy function, and include waxes, phospholipids, cerebrosides, fats, and related or derived compounds.

Lipids provide nine calories per gram ingested – more than twice the energy as carbohydrates and proteins. The lipids grouping includes fats and edible oils such as butter and olive oil, as well as phospholipids, cholesterol, and steroids (all of which have important roles in cell structure and metabolism

Proteins
Proteins – usually referred to as amino acids in terms of nutrition – are the building blocks of life. The body needs proteins to repair and maintain essential structures and functions, because all human body cells contains protein as a major part of the skin, muscles, organs, and glands. Excluding bile and urine, protein is also found in all body fluids. [ix]

Proteins provide four calories per gram ingested. They are made of chains of amino acids, found most readily in meats, fish, eggs, and milk. However, it is not necessary to eat animal products in order to obtain all the necessary protein for a healthy diet. In fact, a high-protein diet could put strain on the kidneys and cause other health problems. Protein can be easily found in soy, beans, legumes, nut butters, and certain types of grain (such as wheat germ). Proteins provide four calories per gram ingested.

Vitamins
Vitamins are organic compounds essential for normal growth and nutrition and are required in small quantities in the diet since they cannot always be synthesized by the body.

Water-soluble
According to the medical dictionary, water-soluble vitamins are not stored in the body in appreciable quantities and are easily excreted in the urine. These vitamins (all vitamins except A, D, E and K) must be ingested regularly as foods or supplements to maintain health. Water-soluble

vitamins assist in essential enzyme activity like energy production from fats and carbohydrates. A deficiency in these vitamins can severely affect rapidly metabolizing tissues in the blood, skin, nervous system, and digestive tract.

Fat-soluble

According to the medical dictionary, fat-soluble vitamins are specifically vitamins A, D, E, and K that are soluble in fat solvents and are absorbed along with dietary fats. These vitamins are not usually excreted in the urine and rather are stored in the liver in moderate amounts. Most individuals do not need vitamin supplements for fat-soluble vitamins. In fact, a buildup or excess of these vitamins can be toxic and lead to health issues.

Nutrition and Exercise Recommendations

On average, a "normal" person should intake no more than 2000 calories per day and should get moderate levels of exercise for **at least** 150 minutes per week – that is, 20 minutes per day or 30 minutes 5 times a week. [xii]

Benefits

There are many benefits of regular exercise and living an active lifestyle besides losing weight and feeling healthier overall. The list below, from the Mayo Clinic, shares a few of these many reasons: [vii]

- Exercise controls weight. Engaging in physical activity makes you burn calories, and the more intense the exercise, the more calories are burned!

- Exercise combats health conditions and diseases. Regular physical activity can help prevent and manage a many health problems or concerns. This concept is explored further in the section below.

- Exercise improves mood. Physical activity stimulates various brain chemicals like epinephrine, serotonin, and dopamine that leave an individual feeling happier and more relaxed.

- Exercise boosts energy. Physical exertion delivers oxygen and nutrients to the body's tissues and helps the cardiovascular system work more efficiently. When the heart and lungs work more efficiently, the body has more energy!

- Exercise promotes better sleep. Regular physical activity can help individuals fall asleep faster and deepen their sleep so they go into a better resting state and feel more refreshed after they wake.

The Role of Exercise in Persons with Chronic Diseases

Living a healthy lifestyle that includes regular physical activity "boosts high-density lipoprotein (HDL), or *good* cholesterol and decreases unhealthy triglycerides. [vii] This process keeps the blood flowing smoothly, which decreases the risk of cardiovascular diseases and other prevalent chronic diseases.

Weight Loss Methods which Do Not Work

Most therapies or methods that promise "rapid weight loss" do not work and are actually bad for the body! One of the most popular and dangerous weight loss methods are starvation diets and Very Low-Calorie diets. These include juice fasts, and so-called "master cleanse diets," that allow intake of only water, lemon juice, maple syrup, and cayenne pepper. These types of diets have been around since at least the 1950s and often promise detoxification through colonics or enemas. [x]

Another popular weight loss method that usually does not work is the use of diet pills and supplements. These supplements claim to speed weight loss, often by blocking absorption of nutrients, increasing metabolism, or burning fat, but in reality they do little or nothing to actually curb hunger or assist in the weight loss process. [x]

Skipping meals to decrease caloric intake is another popular method of dieting which does not work. In fact, studies show that people who skip breakfast are more likely to become obese and overeat than people who eat five to six portioned meals per day. There are many serious health risks to crash dieting including: gallstones, dehydration, malnutrition, electrolyte imbalances, headaches, irritability, fatigue, dizziness, constipation, menstrual irregularities, hair loss, muscle loss, and even death . [x]

In reality, there is no shortcut or method to replace a healthy diet and regular exercise in order to lose weight and be healthy.

Metabolic Rates

According to the Mayo Clinic, metabolism is the process by which the body converts what a person intakes into energy. This complex process combines the calories eaten with oxygen to release energy through ATP that the body needs to function. [vi]

The **resting metabolic rate** is the normal metabolic rate with no external pressure or activity. The **basal metabolic rate** is the measurement of the minimum amount of metabolic activity used to survive and function. This basal metabolic rate is different for each person and is determined based on the following properties: [vi]

- Body size and composition: Larger people with more muscle burn more calories, even at rest.
- Gender: Men have less body fat and more muscle than women of the same age and weight, so they are always burning more calories.
- Age: As people get older, they lose muscle mass and increase fat storage, which slows down calorie burning.

However, the terms Resting Rate and Basal Rate are used interchangeably in the real world, even though they technically are not the same.

Metabolic Processes and Energy Production

The process of creating energy in the human body is called cellular respiration and occurs mostly within the mitochondria, or "power house" of the cell. Humans derive our energy from ATP (Adenosine Triphosphate) which is created by breaking down glucose (which you may recall, comes from carbohydrates). The three major phases of cellular respiration are Glycolysis, the Krebs Cycle, and the Electron Transport Chain.

When glucose is ingested, it goes through these metabolic pathways reacting with substrates in different parts of the body in order to eventually create ATP. One glucose molecule can create between 30-32 ATP. However, we use hundreds of thousands of ATP every day, therefore this process is essential and occurs quickly. The entire reason that humans need to breathe is to enable this aerobic process of creating ATP, so that we can have energy to complete basic tasks and live. ATP production through cellular respiration in the mitochondria is essential to life in living things.

Female Athlete Triad

Female Athlete Triad may sound like an impressive name, but in reality, it describes a trio of serious health problems that commonly occur in female athletes: disordered eating, low bone mass, and amenorrhea (cessation of the menstrual cycle). Society alone reinforces unhealthy and unrealistic expectations for female (and male) body types, but sports which emphasize leanness – such as cross country running, dancing, etc. – are more likely to produce athletes with these conditions.

The following is a list of risk factors associated with this disorder: [i]

- Playing sports that require weight checks.
- Social isolation due to sporting activities.
- Exercising more than necessary for a sport.
- Pressure to "win at all costs."
- Punitive consequences for weight gain.
- Controlling parents and/or coaches[21]

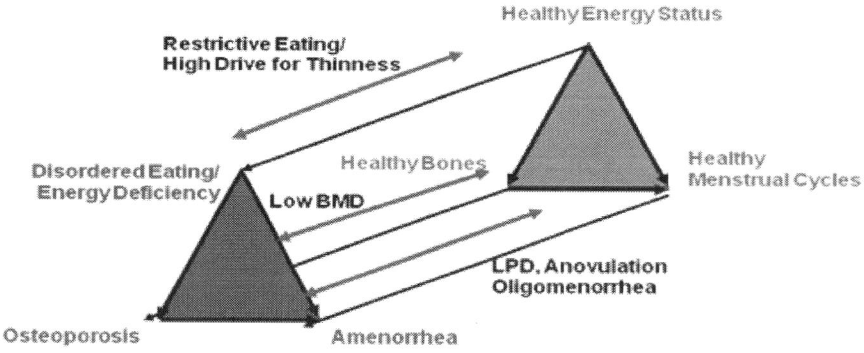

It has been determined that a primary cause of Triad-related health problems, such as menstrual abnormalities and bone loss, is a chronic energy deficiency. The amount that an athlete with this disorder eats is simply not enough to meet the caloric demands of daily exercise training. In other words, energy deficiency occurs when there is a negative imbalance between food intake and energy expenditure through exercise due to an intentional caloric restriction or an increase in exercise.[i]

Most educational efforts aimed at preventing Female Athlete Triad focus on nutrition and eating disorders, but a comprehensive approach should include not only clinically recognized eating disorders, such as anorexia nervosa and bulimia nervosa, but also subclinical disordered eating behaviors, such as

[21] *Image from:* http://www.femaleathletetriad.org/for-athletes-coaches/what-is-the-triad/

caloric restriction. Many athletes, who fail to meet the criteria for an eating disorder, but display a preoccupation with body weight and a poor body image, are part of this subclinical category. [i]

Conversions

During testing, you'll need to be familiar with the following conversions.

Inches to Centimeters

One inch is equivalent to 2.54 centimeters. One centimeter is equivalent to 0.39 inches. For example:

- If you wanted to convert 50 inches into centimeters, you would multiply 50 by 2.54 to get 127 centimeters.
- If you wanted to convert 50 centimeters to inches, you would multiply 50 by 0.39 to get 19.5 inches.

So, 1 in. = 2.54 cm, and 1 cm. = 0.39 in.

Pounds to Kilograms

One pound is equivalent to 0.45 kilograms. One kilogram is equivalent to 2.2 pounds. For example:

- If you wanted to convert 50 pounds into kilograms, you would multiply 50 by 0.45 to get 22.2 kilograms.
- If you wanted to convert 50 kilograms to pounds, you would multiply 50 by 2.2 to get 110 pounds.

So, 1 lb. = 0.45 kg, and1 kg = 2.2 lbs.

Test Your Knowledge: Nutrition and Weight Management

1. How many calories are in one pound? 3,500 calories/pound

2. What are the three most common types of eating disorders? Anorexia, Bulimia, Binge-Eating

3. What is the most abundant compound of the human body besides fat? Water

4. How can two people that weigh the same and are the same height look different? Why? Body Comp.

5. Convert 150 pounds into kilograms. $150 \text{ lbs} \times \frac{1 \text{ kg}}{2.2 \text{ lbs}} =$

6. Convert 30 centimeters into inches. $30 \text{ cm} \times \frac{1 \text{ inch}}{2.54 \text{ cm}} =$

7. Define Waist-to-Hip Ratio.

8. Who should have a higher "normal" body fat percentage – men or women? Why? childbirth

9. Name and define the three major types of macronutrients.

10. What is a vitamin? Why is it important?

11. What are two common ways to measure body fat?

12. What is the new "My Plate" initiative?

Test Your Knowledge: Nutrition and Weight Management – Answers

1. 3, 500 calories per pound.

2. Anorexia Nervosa, Bulimia Nervosa, Binge-Eating Disorder.

3. Water.

4. They have different body compositions; i.e., they can weigh the same, but since muscle weighs more than fat, one person could be more fit than another, even if they have the same height and weight.

5. 67.5 kg (150 * .45 = 67.5).

6. 11.7 (30 * .39 = 11.7).

7. A waist to hip ratio (WHR) is a fraction that represents the circumference of the waist divided by the circumference of the hip.

8. Women have a higher percentage of body fat due to childbearing characteristics.

9. **Carbohydrates:** Carbohydrates are the most important source of energy for the body. The digestive system changes carbohydrates into glucose (blood sugar). The body uses this sugar for energy for cells, tissues, and organs.

Proteins: Proteins are made of chains of amino acids and are the building blocks of life. The body needs proteins to repair and maintain essential structures and functions. Every cell in the human body contains protein. It is a major part of the skin, muscles, organs, and glands. Protein is also found in all body fluids, except bile and urine.

Lipids: Various substances that are not soluble in water and include fats, waxes, phospholipids, cerebrosides, and related or derived compounds.

10. Vitamins are any of a group of organic compounds that are essential for normal growth and nutrition and are required in small quantities in the diet. They are important because they cannot be synthesized by the body and are essential to survival.

11. Skinfold measurements and bioelectric impedance analysis.

12. It is an easier way to visually represent the food pyramid showing how much of each nutrient type you should eat per meal.

References and Additional Reading

This chapter utilized the work of many outside texts, which you may also find useful as supplemental reading materials.

i. Female Athlete Triad. (2012). *What is the triad?* http://www.femaleathletetriad.org/for-athletes-coaches/what-is-the-triad/
ii. Kravitz, L., & Heyward, V. (n.d.). *Getting a grip on body composition.* http://www.unm.edu/~lkravitz/Article folder/underbodycomp.html
iii. Lein, S. (2012). *Types of eating disorders.* http://www.eatingdisordersonline.com/explain/index.php
iv. Mayo Clinic. (2012). *Eating disorders.* http://www.mayoclinic.com/health/eating-disorders/DS00294
v. Mayo Clinic. (2012). *Calories.* http://www.mayoclinic.com/health/calories/WT00011
vi. Mayo Clinic. (2012). *Metabolism.* http://www.mayoclinic.com/health/metabolism/WT00006
vii. Mayo Clinic. (2011). *Exercise: 7 benefits of regular physical activity.* http://www.mayoclinic.com/health/exercise/HQ01676
viii. Medline Plus. (2012). *Carbohydrates.* http://www.nlm.nih.gov/medlineplus/carbohydrates.html
ix. Medline Plus. (2011). *Proteins.* http://www.nlm.nih.gov/medlineplus/ency/article/002467.htm
x. WebMD. (n.d.) *Rapid weight loss.* http://women.webmd.com/pharmacist-11/rapid-weight-loss
xi. World Health Organization. (2011). *Waist circumference and waist-hip ratios.* http://whqlibdoc.who.int/publications/2011/9789241501491_eng.pdf
xii. USDA-US Department of Agriculture. (2012). *Supertracker.* https://www.supertracker.usda.gov/myplan.aspx

Chapter 6: Program Administration, Quality Assurance, and Outcomes Assessment

Program Administration, Quality Assurance, and Outcomes Assessment knowledge are all extremely valuable when planning, implementing, and evaluating the success of a program. Program Administration ensures reduced risk and liability for a successful and profitable program.

Quality Assurance is a process-centered approach to ensuring that a company or organization is providing the best possible products or services to its clientele by planning, programming, and developing a program. Quality Assurance focuses on enhancing and improving the process that is used to create the end result, rather than focusing on the end result itself.

Outcomes Assessment is the ongoing measurable results that are taken from program administration and quality assurance to continue to exceed customer expectations.

Program Development is a systematic process that involves ongoing and structured planning to successfully achieve goals; this includes a needs assessment, informed consent, PAR-Q, business plan, and program planning.

Needs Assessment is a systematic process for determining and addressing needs that may be needed for the improvement in individuals within a community or organization. The needs assessment is a planning process that involves gathering sufficient and appropriate data that will be directed towards developing and implementing a feasible and applicable solution.

The needs assessment data can be collected through surveying the members of the community or organization, collecting health data that is available through local, state, and federal government, or gathering information from services that are already being offered from the community.

A needs assessment is an important part of the planning process when designing a successful program. It can be an effective tool to clarify problems and identify appropriate interventions or solutions. Gathering appropriate and sufficient data informs helps address the group's wants and needs. Needs assessments are only effective when they are ends-focused and provide concrete evidence, which can be used to determine what actions will be most effective and efficient for achieving the desired results.

Informed Consent is an agreement to do something or to allow something to happen, made with complete knowledge of all relevant facts, especially the risks involved. An informed consent will give, in detail, all sufficient information and the expectations of the patient or client in order to allow individuals to make an informed decision about any exercise participation. An informed consent form is not a legal document, but it must still provide all the information to the patient or client about the procedures, limitations, risks, and discomforts, as well as the benefits, of exercise.

Although not a legal document, a facility should use legal counsel in developing informed consent forms, because an informed consent does not provide information on negligence, improper test administration, or insufficient safety procedures. An informed consent does not provide legal immunity to the facility or to the patient or client, but it does provide evidence that the patient or client has been made aware of the procedures, purpose, and risks associated with the test or exercise program.

Information must be provided to the patient in a timely manner and in accordance with the accepted standard of practice among members of the profession with similar training and experience. The patient should be given verbal explanation of the consent form and be able to read and sign the document in a quiet, private setting. The patient should be given an opportunity to ask any questions regarding his or her consent, the informed consent form should be signed and dated, and a copy of the informed consent form should be given to the patient.

A health care professional or personal trainer may be legally liable if a patient or client does not give informed consent for a medical procedure or exercise program and it results in harm to the patient or client, *even if the procedure is properly performed.*

The physical activity readiness questionnaire **(PAR-Q)** is a self-screening tool that can be used by anyone who is planning to start an exercise program. It is often used by health fitness professionals to determine the safety or possible risk of exercise for an individual, based upon the individual's answers to specific health history questions. Being physically active is very safe for most people; however, some people should check with their doctors before they increase their current level of activity.

The PAR-Q has been designed to identify the small number of adults for whom physical activity may be inappropriate or those who should have medical advice concerning the type of activity most suitable for them. This questionnaire can be used for any individual who is ready to start a physical activity program in a health and fitness setting. Clients should read and complete PAR-Q forms in a quiet setting. When they have completed the PAR-Q form, health fitness professionals should review the responses with them to determine health risk status.

A business plan is another important part of program development. This plan gives a detailed description of the facility's mission statement, goals, objectives, program description, financial expenses, and a marketing plan to organize a successful program.

A business plan should always include information regarding any strengths, weaknesses, opportunities, and threats (SWOT) of the services or products being offered by the facility.

The bottom line for any successful business plan is customer service. Without customer service an organization can fail, because the product, health, is not delivering its full potential to the clients. This can adversely affect the business, because these clients may choose not to refer you in the future.

Program Planning is an important and valuable thought process, taking into account various factors such as the needs of the target population, the existing or needed expertise of the care deliverers, and the market demand for particular services. The health and fitness industry is always changing; keep up with these changing trends and modify programs accordingly.

Expertise of the staff or care deliverers is a vital component in the development of program planning. When existing staff are unqualified or underprepared to deliver or do not customarily provide the level of care needed, the business will need to contract labor or services to meet the customer or patient needs (e.g. exercise physiologists, physicians, registered dieticians). An identified market demand is strong justification for offering a particular program or service, because the likelihood of acceptance and ultimately, financial success, is high. Identifying and projecting needs of the clientele is an important and, critical factor in program planning. Program planning sets priorities and establishes effective outcomes.

Case Study Example

Here is a specific case study, similar to one which you may see on the exam. Pay attention to the details, and try to think of a solution before you read the appropriate response.

A new client/patient comes into your facility looking to hire you on as a personal trainer for weight loss, lowering blood pressure, lowering cholesterol, decreasing his A1C levels (blood glucose) and, overall, increase his energy levels.

The patient is 55 years old and very sedentary. Patient has not exercised in over 20 years and is looking to improve his health. Patient is obese and has metabolic syndrome (three or more risk factors for heart disease and stroke). Patient brings in his medical records from his doctor so the personal trainer can review all of his information to start an exercise program. The health fitness professional notices that the information brought in is missing his glucose levels and some of his cholesterol information. LDL cholesterol is the bad cholesterol that increases the risk for atherosclerosis by binding to the arterial walls. High levels of LDL increase heart disease. HDL cholesterol is the good cholesterol that can help remove the LDL cholesterol from the arterial walls, so higher levels are desirable. Glucose levels are important in designing an exercise program due to how exercise, food, and possible diabetes medications will affect the levels of the blood sugar after the exercise program.

<u>Patient Information</u>

55 year old Caucasian male with the following medical history and risk factor profile:

1. <u>Diabetes</u>: He has had type 2 diabetes for the past 6 years.
   He currently takes the following medications:
   - Glucophage (metformin hydrochloride) - two 1000 mg tabs at breakfast and at dinner.
   - Crestor (Rosuvastatin) one 20 mg tablet in the morning.
   - Zestril (Lisinopril) - one 40 mg tablet in the morning.

2. <u>Hypertension</u>: He has a history of stage 1 hypertension : 160/92.

3. <u>High density lipoprotein (HDL)</u> – (unknown)

4. <u>Low density lipoprotein (LDL)</u> – (unknown)

5. <u>Total cholesterol</u> (TC) – 280.

6. <u>Blood sugar</u> – (unknown)

7. <u>Weight</u>: 286 lbs. $\times \frac{1\text{ kg}}{2.2\text{ lbs}} =$

8. <u>Height</u>: 5' 10".

9. <u>Lifestyle</u>: Sedentary.

Smoker: Not mentioned =

Now consider the case:

> Metabolic syndrome is a contradiction to exercise but even though a risk factor, exercise benefits will outweigh these risks. All of the client's medical information should be up to date before starting an exercise program, because liability that can be held against the personal trainer and the facility. The patient should read and sign an informed consent form to let them know all the sufficient information about the participation of the exercise program. The patient signing the informed consent form will bypass the insufficient information needed from the medical chart until it is up to date.
>
> A client or patient with any risk stratification must be identified to determine the participant eligibility before starting an exercise program. The glucose and cholesterol information that is missing from the client's medical chart is important, but not enough to not start an exercise regime. The health fitness professional needs to understand that these blood tests show the patient's health status and will help the professional design an appropriate exercise program.
>
> To start an exercise program, all program components must be established in order for clients to proceed with an exercise plan. A client's exercise prescription should be reflected on all of the patient's medical information and should be followed closely by the health and fitness team.

Business Budgeting is an extremely important part of program planning, which helps control the finances of a company; without financial and budgetary considerations the future of the business can be out of control. Every budget needs strategic planning in order to build a successful business. Accountants usually handle all expenses, evaluate program financial performance, determine program viability, and identify variances to projections, responding accordingly.

Business budgeting should always be realistic, clearly defined, and easily measured. Business budgeting will produce program revenue by billing patients and clients, contracting services for specific client groups and managed care organizations, managing the sale of any merchandise, and qualifying for grants, services, or programs from educational, governmental, or any other foundations. Business budgeting financial and budgetary considerations also include program expenses. These expenses are:

1. **Capital expenses** are usually large, durable items with an extended useful life greater than three years which cost over $1,000. Examples: furniture, exercise equipment, etc.

2. **Noncapital expenses** are day-to-day operational expenses. Examples: supplies, minor equipment, forms, stationary, etc.

Fixed expenses are typically unchanged from month to month, such as rent, payroll, maintenance agreement, etc. **Variable expenses** are based on utilization, including disposable supplies, per diem staff payroll, contract labor, and so forth.

Business administration is the process of managing a business, so that it remains stable and continues to grow. This consists of a number of areas, ranging from operations to management. Most companies have a dedicated group of administrators. The main areas incorporated into business administration are operations, logistics, marketing, economics, Human Resources (HR), and management. An administrator oversees these parts of an organization to make sure that they all function properly and efficiently individually, and that they're all working together to make the business profitable. Administrators also come up with ways to make the department more profitable, and often delegates tasks to employees within departments.

The **Principle of Specificity** states that health fitness training should be relevant and appropriate to the sport for which the individual is training, in order to produce a training effect.

Legal and Ethical Considerations
Health fitness professionals need to take into account legal and ethical considerations when working with clients. A health fitness professional's job is to design exercise programs for their clients; under no circumstance should he or she try to treat or diagnose a medical condition that they think their client may have. Health fitness professionals should have knowledge of legal and ethical considerations and take them seriously when providing care or exercise guidance to their clients, so they can be protected by the law.

Health fitness professionals should always conduct health risk assessments to find out about any underlying health problems their clients might be facing before starting an exercise program. They should always give their clients a written statement of the facilities standards of care, and provide their clients with confidentiality.

Conducting a health **risk assessment** has several potential benefits including identifying health risk factors, controlling health care costs, predicting employee absenteeism, encouraging individuals to take a proactive stance when it comes to personal health care, and monitoring the health status of the general population. Each of these factors can contribute to preventing future health problems. Health risk assessments can reduce health risks and motivate people to make changes to promote better health. When people know that certain lifestyle choices and factors within their control could cause serious illnesses in the future, they are often motivated to start making healthy changes within their lives.

A standard of care is a written statement describing the rules, actions, or conditions that direct patient care. Standards of care guide practice and can be used to evaluate performance. These standards of care must be provided in a facility's programs, policies, and procedures. A standard of care will follow guidelines and protocols that experts would agree with as most appropriate, or "best practice." For instance, a clinic that includes healthcare professionals such as exercise physiologists, respiratory therapists, nurses, etc., should take into account all standards for care for all involved professions. Standards of care are developed in a number of ways; sometimes they are simply developed over time, while sometimes they are the result of clinical findings.

Confidentiality has legal protection when disclosing any private information or secrets discussions between a health fitness professional and a client. An example of confidentiality would be between a doctor and a patient. Any information disclosed to the doctor by the patient should be kept secret, preventing the doctor from sharing this information with anyone else. Health Insurance Portability and Accountability Act (HIPPA) was created to prevent clinical settings, healthcare facilities, health plans, and healthcare providers from sharing a patient's personal information with any other person besides the patient. The Health Insurance Portability and Accountability Act (HIPPA) has established national standards to protect patients by keeping their information and medical records secured.

Tort Laws offer remedies to individuals harmed by the unreasonable actions of others. A tort is a type of a civil wrong doing, whether that tort is intentional or if negligence is involved. An intentional tort is usually an offence committed by someone to intentionally harm someone else. A negligence tort is more often seen in an education or healthcare setting. A negligence tort is an act leading to injury that is neither expected nor intended. A negligence tort is seen more often in a healthcare setting because injury should never be intended or expected.

An example of a negligence tort would be a health fitness professional spotting his client with a bar bell chest press exercise:

> The client tries to press the bar bell back up, but the health fitness professional is not paying attention and the bar bell smashes down on the client's chest. The health fitness professional never intended or expected for his client to get hurt, but by not paying attention to his client while the lift was taking place, he did injure the client, who had to go to the hospital.

Three factors must be established in every tort action. These three factors are:

1. The defendant owed the claimant a duty of care.
2. The defendant breached that duty of care.
3. Reasonably foreseeable damage was caused by the breach of duty.

Remedies for tortious acts usually involve paying the client an amount of money for the negligence that occurred. If an injury occurred, the negligence case could go to civil court or be settled out of court.

The difference between negligence and malpractice is that **negligence** is an unintentional failure to exercise a generally excepted standard resulting in harm or injury to someone, while **malpractice** is a specific type of negligence that usually involves claims against a licensed professional who fails to provide services that are written in the standard of care, subsequently causing harm or injury to the client or patient.

Four Factors which must be present to demonstrate professional negligence or malpractice:

1. Proximate Cause shows that the client suffered harm due to breach of duty.
2. Damages are being sought from the harm that was caused to the client.
3. Duty is a legal obligation from a licensed professional that was not performed.
4. Breach of duty shows that the licensed professional did not perform this duty.

A **duty** is a legal obligation, something that someone else is supposed to do under contract. Health fitness professionals must be aware of their legal obligations and responsibilities when it comes to negligence, malpractice, liability insurance, the use of the medical and testing procedures, informed consent, and the authority for exercise prescription.

Health fitness professionals have four basic duties by which they should abide:

1. Inform.
2. Instruct.
3. Monitor.
4. Supervise.

Waivers are forms that health fitness professionals have their clients sign to limit their liability. Waivers are highly recommended for every client who is going to begin an exercise program, because they can prevent or limit the likelihood of lawsuits arising from negligence. In many instances, waivers are very effective in limiting liability attributable to personal negligence. Waivers can be created by the health fitness professional, but should always be reviewed by an attorney to ensure they conform to state laws.

There are certain legal claims which CANNOT be waived; these claims are safety requirements such as CPR Qualifications, gross misconduct, and intentional misconduct.

Test Your Knowledge: Program Administration, Quality Assurance, and Outcomes Assessment

1. What is considered a tort law?
   a) Negligence tort.
   b) Bad tort.
   c) Free will tort.
   d) Duty tort.

2. True/False: Malpractice is a type of negligence.

3. True/False: Health fitness professionals should have their clients sign waivers.

4. True/False: Informed consent is a legal form that protects health fitness professionals from liability lawsuits.

5. Which of the following statements best describe non-capital budgets?
   a) They are not necessary with exercise programs.
   b) They are included in standard of care form.
   c) They include costs of supplies, minor equipment, forms and stationary.
   d) The principle of specificity.

6. True/False: HIPPA protects a patient or client's confidentiality.

7. Describe a duty.

8. What are the four basic duties of a health fitness professional?

9. Which of the following statements concerning needs assessments is true?
   a) They are no help with the evaluation of a program.
   b) They are useful for marketing purposes.
   c) The needs assessment is a planning process that involves gathering sufficient and appropriate data, which will be directed towards developing and implementing a feasible and applicable solution.
   d) They are used to make management happy.

10. What is a PAR-Q form used for?
   a) It is a legal form.
   b) Budget assessment.
   c) Self-screening tool.
   d) Policies and procedures.

Test Your Knowledge: Program Administration, Quality Assurance, and Outcomes Assessment – Answers

1. **a)** A negligence tort is the most common tort seen in an education or healthcare setting. A negligence tort is an act leading to injury that is neither expected nor intended.

2. **a)** Negligence is an unintentional failure to exercise a generally excepted standard, causing harm or injury to someone Malpractice is a type of negligence.

3. **a)** Waivers are a form that a personal trainer should have their client sign to limit their liability. Waivers are highly recommended for every client who is going to begin an exercise program, because they can prevent or limit the likelihood of lawsuits arising from negligence

4. **b) Informed Consent** is an agreement to do something or to allow something to happen, made with complete knowledge of all relevant facts, such as the risks involved. An informed consent will give in detail sufficient information and the expectations of the patient or client to make an informed decision about any exercise participation.

   An informed consent form is not a legal document, but it has to provide all the information to the patient or client about the procedures, limitations, risks, and discomforts, as well as the benefits, of exercise.

5. **c) Noncapital expenses** are day-to-day operational expenses such as supplies, minor equipment, forms, and stationary.

6. **a)** The Health Insurance Portability and Accountability Act (HIPPA) was created to protect patients. It prevents clinical settings, healthcare facilities, health plans, and healthcare providers from sharing patient information with anyone besides the patient.

7. **A duty** is a legal obligation, something that someone else is supposed to do under contract.

8. There are four basic duties that they should abide by: Inform, Instruct, Monitor, and Supervise.

9. **c) Needs Assessment** is a systematic process for determining and addressing needs that may be needed for the improvement in individuals within a community or organization. The needs assessment is a planning process that involves gathering sufficient and appropriate data that will be directed towards developing and implementing a feasible and applicable solution.

10. **c)** The physical activity readiness questionnaire **(PAR-Q)** is a self-screening tool that can be used by anyone who is planning to start an exercise program. It is often used by fitness trainers or coaches to determine the safety or possible risk of exercising for an individual based upon their answers to specific health history questions.

Chapter 7: Safety, Injury Prevention, and Emergency Procedures

RISKS OF EXERCISE

For most healthy people, the benefits of exercise far outweigh the risks. However, even for those populations which are healthy and active, potential risks still exist when engaging in physical activity. As a professional, you should understand the potential of those risks, the most common being:

1. **Overuse Injuries**: Occur when the body has been taxed beyond its capabilities. Remind your clients that being healthy and well means treating their bodies well; this includes exercising, of course, but also learning to realize when the body needs rest. Common overuse injuries are muscle pulls, sprains, and strains.

2. **Over-exertion**: These injuries are similar to overuse injuries in that both occur when the body has been pushed beyond its capabilities. Over-exertion may result in exhaustion, shortness of breath, dizziness, and other dangerous conditions.

3. **Accidents**: It is important to always pay close attention to clients in order to create the safest environment possible; however, you should always be prepared for the "human element" of physical exertion. These can include dropped equipment, improper form, inadequate spacing which results in collision between bodies, etc. – resulting in accidental injury.

4. **Prior Health Conditions and Injuries**: When a client has a history of injuries or health conditions, they are more likely to be at risk for future ones. It is important for you, as the professional, to be made aware of any and all existing conditions. There is nothing sneaky about finding out about existing conditions; simply asking before commencing a program. For example, you could say, "If anyone has any health conditions or injuries, let me know before we begin." You can even go around before beginning, if you have the time, and speak individually with each client, introducing yourself and ascertaining their individual fitness needs.

All of these risks, and those less-common, can be exacerbated by many factors, including:

- When the exercise is particularly vigorous, as in extreme or competitive sports.

- When training is occurring under adverse conditions, as in high altitudes, extremely hot or cold climates, or outside climates which consist of rocky or uneven ground.

- An existing history of health conditions (obesity, impaired glucose tolerance, elevated HDL, elevated blood pressure, and/or a family history of any of the above).

- Clients who drink or smoke.

Though uncommon, strenuous exercise can even result in sudden death in non-athletic, teenage, and young adult athletes with inherited cardiac disorders, as well as in older adults with risk factors for coronary heart disease.

Cardiopulmonary and Metabolic Conditions

Some of the more common medical conditions are cardiopulmonary and metabolic conditions, such as diabetes, hyperglycemia, hypoglycemia, and cardiac arrhythmias.

Diabetes

As discussed in previous chapters, diabetes is one of the leading causes of death in the United States, and those with diabetes can experience serious complications during physical activity. Exercise is often prescribed to prevent and control diabetes; however, those with diabetes can experience serious complications during physical activity.

Diabetes' full name is **diabetes mellitus**, which defines a group of diseases which alter how the body uses blood glucose (blood sugar). Glucose is an important source of energy for the body, fueling cells which make up muscles and tissues, providing the fuel for metabolism, and acting as the primary source of fuel for the brain. There are two types of diabetes:

- **Type 1** diabetes (insulin dependent diabetes) typically occurs in people under the age of 40 and is a chronic condition in which the pancreas produces little or no insulin.

- **Type 2** diabetes (insulin resistant) occurs when the body becomes resistant to the effects of insulin or fails to produce enough insulin. This is the more common form of diabetes.

It is important to learn if any of your clients have either type of diabetes. However, be aware that many people may not wish to share personal conditions for some personal reason. Stress the importance of learning these details and offer several means for your clients to communicate this information with you privately, via email, phone, or office consultations.

Once you become aware of a client with diabetes, you should provide and make sure clients follow these general safety guidelines:

- Know the ideal blood glucose level. (Between 100 – 200mg/dL, one to two hours after eating.)

- Regulate glucose levels by timing workout sessions in relation to meals and insulin dosage.

- Check blood glucose levels before and after workouts.

- Clients should consult their physicians regarding the possibility of reducing insulin by 10% to 50% when beginning an exercise program, due to pronounced effect which exercise has on insulin production.

- Perform a proper warm-up and cool-down.

- Wear appropriate footwear.

- Remain hydrated.

- Avoid exercising in extreme conditions.

Hyperglycemia
Diabetes is not the only condition which effects blood glucose. **Hyperglycemia** means that a person has high blood glucose. ("Hyper" means "high," or "above.") Since the ideal blood glucose level is between 100 and 200 mg/dL; a hyperglycemic body will have a glucose level that exceeds 200 mg/dL.

Some people constantly have high blood glucose, and they should inform you of this condition. However, hyperglycemia can occur in healthy populations as well, due to a sudden change in diet or body composition. In either case, both you and your clients should be aware of the symptoms and treatments of hyperglycemia.

Symptoms associated with hyperglycemia:

1. Frequent urination.
2. Increased thirst.
3. Blurred vision.
4. Fatigue.
5. Headache.
6. Cardiac arrhythmia.
7. Deep and rapid breathing.

If you notice any of these symptoms, and suspect that a client has become hyperglycemic, you should:

1. Give the client water.
2. If possible, have the client test their blood sugar levels.
3. Once the client knows the client's blood sugar level, have him or her take the dosage of insulin prescribed by his or her doctor. If the client does not have an insulin prescription, seek medical attention immediately.

Hypoglycemia
On the other side of the spectrum is **hypoglycemia**, which means low blood glucose, specifically a glucose level below 70 mg/dL. (A good way to remember the difference between "hyper" and "hypo" is through rhyming: "hypo" rhymes with "low.")

Symptoms associated with hypoglycemia:

- Shakiness.
- Dizziness.
- Sweating.

- Hunger.
- Irritability or moodiness.
- Anxiety or nervousness.
- Headache.
- Confusion.
- Pallid skin.

Just as with hyperglycemia, even healthy populations ought to be aware of the possibilities of becoming hypoglycemic.

If a client shows symptoms of hypoglycemia, health fitness professionals should:

- Stop the workout.
- Have the client sit or lie down.
- If they are able to check their glucose levels, have them do so.
- Raise the blood glucose levels immediately with a rapidly absorbing carbohydrate such as a piece of candy or fruit juice. **Avoid diet soft drinks, as they have no sugar.*
- If the client has a glucose gel or tablet, he or she can take this instead of a carbohydrate.
- Insist the client rest until signs of improvement occur.
- Check the client's blood glucose levels when they start to feel better.
- A blood glucose level of 100 mg/dL is acceptable to resume activity.
- If the client shows little to no signs of improvement, seek medical attention immediately.

Cardiac Arrhythmias: Cardiopulmonary Conditions
Cardiac arrhythmias, or heart rhythm abnormalities, happen when the heart does not pump properly, which causes it to beat too fast or too slow. Though most arrhythmias are harmless and may be reduced by regular exercise, serious problems can sometimes occur during physical activity. [22]

[22] To see animated visuals of heart arrhythmias, refer to the American Heart Association's® "Watch, Learn, and Live" Interactive Cardiovascular Library.

Bradycardia
Bradycardia is a condition wherein the heart has an abnormally slow heart rate, which is less than 60 beats per minute. This can result in the following symptoms:

- Fainting.
- Dizziness.
- Lightheadedness.
- Fatigue.
- Shortness of breath.
- Angina.
- Confusion.
- Tiring quickly during exercise.

If a client shows symptoms of bradycardia, health fitness professionals should:

1. Stop the workout.
2. Perform CPR, if needed.
3. Seek medical attention immediately.

Tachycardia
Bradycardia has an opposite condition: tachycardia. **Tachycardia** is when the heart has an abnormally *fast* rate, exceeding 100 beats per minute. Tachycardia may produce no symptoms, but extreme cases can lead to unconsciousness, stroke, and sudden cardiac arrest. These are serious, dangerous conditions, and you should be aware of the following symptoms:

- Dizziness.
- Lightheadedness.
- Palpitations.
- Angina.
- Shortness of breath.

If a client shows symptoms of tachycardia, health fitness professionals should:

1. Stop the workout.
2. Perform CPR, if needed.
3. Seek medical attention immediately.

EMERGENCY SITUATIONS

Health fitness professionals are responsible for client safety, and while prevention should be practiced, you must also be prepared to respond appropriately should an emergency arise. Health fitness professionals who work in health clubs should familiarize themselves with their company's emergency procedures, while independent health fitness professionals should develop their own written plans of action.

Controlling an Emergency Situation

In the case of controlling emergency situations, the best offense is a good defense. Have a plan in mind to prevent emergencies from happening in the first place, and have a backup plan prepared in case those emergencies occur anyway.

Prevention
Health fitness professionals should provide adequate instruction and supervision when working with clients.

> For example, a client who is using the treadmill for the first time should be instructed to stand on the runners of the treadmill (straddling the belt) and to hold onto the hand rails before activating the treadmill. This will prevent the client from being taken off guard and being injured when the belt starts to move.

Health fitness professionals must also ensure that all equipment in their facility is regularly inspected, well maintained, and safe for usage. Faulty equipment is an injury waiting to happen.

During an exercise session, pay close attention to each of your clients and keep an eye out for any complications. Stop the exercise session immediately if a client can no longer speak or experiences any of the following: pain, discomfort, nausea, dizziness, lightheadedness, chest pain, an irregular heartbeat, shortness of breath, and/or unusual fatigue.

Emergency Preparedness
A well-prepared health fitness professional reviews his or her clients' medical profiles to ensure as much knowledge about clients as possible.

> For example, if a client indicates on the medical history form that they are diabetic, the health fitness professional should then follow up with appropriate questions, potentially request a doctor's consent, and design workouts accordingly, monitoring the client at all times.

Health fitness professionals should also know the steps necessary in a medical emergency.

> For example, should a diabetic emergency occur the health fitness professional should call 911, provide adequate care for any life-threatening situations, and give juice or candy to the client or have them take their glucose pill until help arrives.

To further prepare for emergency situations, make sure that you know the appropriate laws for exercise and emergency medical aid within your state and that you maintain the necessary level of insurance as required by your state. Research current industry trends for emergency treatments, and keep your CPR, AED, and Basic Life Support certifications up-to-date.

Clients should have current and accurate PAR-Q forms and medical records on-file, as well as emergency contact numbers. Have the following items nearby and easily accessible: phone numbers for emergency responders and emergency medical devices (CPR micro-shield, first aid kit, AED, etc.). Always plan to follow-up after an emergency within a reasonable time frame.

General Emergency Response Guidelines
Despite your planning and preventative measures, emergencies can always arise. When they do, your preparedness can make all the difference in a critical situation. Knowing how to respond in an emergency can save a person's life, and the faster one responds, the better. Practice can be very helpful to ensure that an emergency is handled calmly and effectively. The following pages detail general guidelines for responding to emergency situations.

Responding to a Seizure

1. Call 911.
2. Lower the person to the ground, on their side if possible.
3. Protect the head from injury by placing a cushion underneath or gently holding it.
4. Turn the person's head to the side.
5. If possible, cover the person's body with a blanket to preserve dignity (some people may lose control of their bowels and/or bladder when seizing).
6. When seizure has ended, place person in recovery position.
7. Check their breathing and pulse.
8. Address any injuries.
9. Comfort the person.

Responding to Shock

1. Monitor the person's breathing and pulse.
2. Keep the person warm.
3. Address any external bleeding.
4. Elevate the legs about 12 inches to maintain circulation. **Avoid doing so if the person is nauseated or having difficulty breathing, may have a neck, head or back injury or potential broken bones, or if moving the person will cause more pain.*
5. Avoid giving the person anything to drink.

Responding to External Bleeding

1. Apply pressure.
2. Apply a bandage.
3. Call 911.
4. Monitor the person's breathing and pulse.

Responding to Choking

1. Call 911.
2. Support the person and lean them forward.
3. Render 5 back blows with the heel of your hand.
4. Administer the Heimlich Maneuver. Make a fist and grab it with the other hand. Put the thumb side of your fist against the person's stomach, just above the navel. Administer 5 thrusts to the abdomen.
5. Continue until the object is forced out or the person is able to breathe or cough on their own.

Responding to Diabetic Emergency

1. Address any life-threatening emergencies.
2. If they are conscious, give the person fruit juice, non-diet soda, or candy.
3. If the person is conscious, but does not feel better approximately five minutes after taking sugar, call 911 immediately.
4. If the person is unconscious, call 911 immediately.

Musculoskeletal Injuries

Muscle strains, sprains, fractures, joint dislocations and general muscle pain are common injuries that often vary in severity. Administering at-home treatment at the onset of such injuries is fairly simple and usually effective depending on the injury's severity.

It is important to note that if severe trauma is suffered medical attention should be sought immediately.

In the case of early injury treatment, remember the acronym **R.I.C.E. (Rest, Ice, Compression, and Elevation)**:

Rest: Reduce or stop using the injured area for 48 hours. Leg injuries, may require complete rest.

Ice: Apply ice to the injured area for 20 minutes at a time, 4 to 8 times per day. A cold pack, ice bag, or a plastic bag filled with crushed ice can be used.

Compression: Compression may help to reduce swelling. Seek medical advice to determine the best option but those most commonly used are bandages such as elastic wraps, special boots, air casts, and splints.

Elevation: Elevate the injured area above the level of the heart. Pillows, for example, can be used to help elevate an injured limb.

Proper Documentation and Informed Consent

Health fitness professionals should use informed consent documents to ensure that clients fully understand the inherent risks of engaging in a training program. These consent forms allow clients to make informed decisions to proceed, while protecting health fitness professionals from liability for injuries that may occur from inherent and treatment risks of the training program.

It is important to note that a waiver is still necessary to avoid being liable for injuries that result from negligence. Health fitness professions should review these documents in detail with their clients, so that an informed decision can be made before both parties agree to move forward. Both the informed consent form and the waiver should comply with state law. Signed consent forms and waivers should be kept on file at all times.

Key Components for an Informed Consent Form should include:

- The name of the health fitness business.
- Clearly list program objectives, benefits, and risks.
- Specify whether or not a physician's consent is required to start the training program or if it is clients' responsibility to do so on their own.

Key Components for a Liability Waiver should include:

- The name of the health fitness business.
- List any and all potential activities that the training program will include.
- The state where the waiver is being utilized.
- A clear statement regarding the assumption of risk.

CREATING SAFE ENVIRONMENTS

The American Disabilities Act
Health fitness professionals who own their own fitness studios are required by the ADA to improve accessibility to those with disabilities. While the ADA does not force small businesses to take on excessive expenses that could be detrimental to the business, small businesses that serve the public must remove physical "barriers" that are "readily achievable," based on their size and the economic means of the business.

> For example, small businesses that offer public parking must also provide designated accessible parking spaces that are closest to the entrance. Most entrances to businesses use 36 inch wide doors that are wide enough to be accessible.

A review of training areas, lounges, locker rooms, restrooms, showers, and counter space should be done to ensure reasonable access for all. Facilities should make every effort to welcome and accommodate those with disabilities.

How to Create a Safe Environment in the Facility You Work In
Maintaining a safe environment for clients is imperative. A great deal of injuries and accidents occur from improper use of equipment and lack of supervision. Promoting safe practices, providing safe equipment, and supervising activity are all good measures towards creating a safe fitness facility.

Tips for creating a safe fitness facility:

- Maintain a clean facility, and encourage workers and clients to do the same by keeping cleaning wipes and/or sanitizer in plain view.
- Only trained professional should assemble and test exercise equipment prior to use.
- Allow at least 100 square feet of training space for each individual using an area at any given time.
- Inspect and clean equipment regularly; remove any damaged equipment promptly.
- Utilize visuals to describe appropriate usage of equipment.
- Ensure that everyone employed by the facility has current fitness certifications and current CPR certifications.
- Never allow clients to utilize the facility without supervision.
- Encourage clients to bring a small hand towel when working out.

The Importance of the Warm-Up and Cool-Down

Warm-ups and cool-downs are essential for any workout. They are often overlooked and undervalued, however, by clients who are short on time or focused on specific fitness goals.

Warm-Up
The warm-up does not necessarily prevent injury, as was once commonly thought, but it is believed to enhance overall performance. A good warm-up should always be the prerequisite for any physical activity. It helps to ease the body into exercise by gradually raising the body temperature, increasing blood flow, and preparing the body for more vigorous activity.

The warm-up should be 5 to 10 minutes in duration and include:

- Low intensity, cardiovascular activity that resembles activities planned for the workout.
- Stretching of all major muscle groups.

Cool-Down
The cool-down accomplishes the function of transitioning the body from a state of vigorous activity back into a normal resting mode. This critical transition phase prevents blood from pooling in the lower extremities, which can lead to dizziness and/or fainting. The cool-down should have the opposite effect of the warm-up. The heart rate will gradually decrease and the body temperature will lower.
Benefits of the cool-down include: improving flexibility, removing lactic acid, reducing the onset of muscle soreness, and allowing the cardio respiratory system to adequately recuperate from the heighten state of activity.

Flexibility exercises should be incorporated into the cool-down phase, which will cause the body to relax through corrective stretching and prevent the buildup of lactic acid that leads to muscle soreness. Good options for flexibility include static stretches or myofascial release.

Absolute and Relative Contraindications with Exercise Testing and Training

While exercise is generally beneficial, there are those for whom exercise could be deadly. In such cases, physical activity or a training program is not recommended. There are also cases wherein close supervision by a medical professional is necessary.

Absolute contraindications can be defined as permanent or temporary restrictions that may be lifted once the condition is effectively treated, stabilized or past the acute stage. They prohibit one from engaging in all or, in some cases, certain types of physical activity until the condition has improved and it is safe to exercise. These are cases wherein the risks of exercise clearly outweigh the benefits.

Examples of absolute contraindications to exercise testing:

- Acute myocardial infarction.
- Unstable angina.
- Uncontrolled cardiac arrhythmias that cause symptoms.
- Symptomatic severe aortic stenosis.
- Uncontrolled heart failure.

- Acute pulmonary embolus or pulmonary infarction.
- Acute myocarditis or pericarditis.
- Acute aortic dissection.
- Left main coronary stenosis.
- Moderate stenotic valvular heart disease.
- Electrolyte abnormalities.
- Severe arterial hypertension.
- Tachyarrhythmias or bradyarrhythmias.
- Hypertrophic cardiomyopathy and other forms of obstruction.
- Mental or physical impairment leading to inability to exercise safely.
- High-degree atrioventricular block.
- Acute infectious disease.
- Inability to obtain a doctor's consent.

Relative Contraindications tend to be highly variable. In such cases, the value of exercise testing or a training program may exceed any risk. There may still be some activities that are restricted, and medical supervision may be required to ensure safety.

- Left main coronary stenosis or its equivalent.
- Moderate stenotic valvular heart disease.
- Electrolyte abnormalities.
- Tachyarrhythmias or bradyarrhythmias.
- Atrial fibrillation with uncontrolled ventricular rate.
- Hypertrophic cardiomyopathy.
- Mental impairment leading to inability to cooperate.
- High-degree AV block.

SPECIFIC KNOWLEDGE

Those with Osteoporosis and Lower Back Pain
Some clients have special prescriptive conditions. Generally speaking, it is they can and should exercise but they may need to do so with limitations and avoid specific activities that may put them at greater risk than the average individual. Such clients need training programs that are geared towards their needs and limitations. They may require medical supervision, as well.

For clients with low back pain, maintaining proper form and correct posture are important. Avoid potentially adverse activities that compromise the spine and neck such as violent twisting, extreme flexion or extension.

Those with osteoporosis or low bone density must also take special care. Since these clients have a higher risk of bone fracture, avoid exercises like pushups, vertical jumps, and vertical trunk flexion. A low impact weight bearing or resistance training program in recommended.

Before you leave this section, take the time to study and understand the following subjects:

Effects of Training on Healthy People
It is no secret that regular exercise helps with physical, mental and social outcomes. In fact, more doctors are prescribing exercise regimens to combat common conditions such as obesity, hypertension, high cholesterol, diabetes, depression, and more. Regular exercise helps maintain a healthy weight and reduce stress. Aerobic exercise can decrease the risk of heart disease by 20 to 60 percent, depending on the exertion level, duration and frequency.

Short Term Effects of Exercise:

- Increased energy and improved insulin action.
- Increased cardiac output.
- Endorphin release.
- Increased metabolism.
- Stress and anxiety reduction.
- Better sleep.

Long Term Effects of Exercise:

- Weight loss.
- Mobility.
- Disease prevention.

Types of Stretching

Stretching may help improve flexibility, which may also improve athletic performance and lower the risk of injury. **Flexibility** is important when engaging in physical activities, because it helps the joints move through their full range of motion.

> For example, a tight Achilles tendon can lead to tendonitis over time. Stretching the Achilles tendon, however, can improve the range of motion in the ankle and, therefore, decrease the risk of micro trauma to the tendon that can lead to overload and injury.

Stretching also increases the blood flow to muscles which is critical before engaging in vigorous activity.

There are 3 types of stretches:

1. **Ballistic (Dynamic) Stretching**: A method of stretching wherein bouncing is incorporated into the stretch. The final position is not held. This is not an ideal method of stretching.

2. **Active Stretching**: A method of stretching that uses agonist (contracting) and antagonist (opposing) muscles. When the agonist muscle contract, it inhibits the contraction of the opposing antagonist muscle. One muscle contracts and the other relaxes. Nerve endings monitor the rate of change and the change in length of the muscles to prevent injury. This protective reaction can make holding the stretch more challenging.

3. **Passive Stretching**: A method of stretching that involves only non-contractile elements (ligaments, fascia, bursae, dura mater, and nerve roots). Examples of this type of stretch are when the muscle is handled physically, such as during therapeutic massage or during isometric exercises in which there is no range of motion of the body part involved.

Avoid bouncing during the stretch. Doing so can result in small tears in the muscle. These tears leave scar tissue as the muscle heals, which tightens the muscle even further, decreasing flexibility and can produce pain. It is recommended that stretches be held for at least 30 seconds to be beneficial.

Test Your Knowledge: Safety, Injury Prevention, and Emergency Procedures

True/False:

1. Hyperglycemia can be defined as low blood sugar.

2. Blurred vision is a symptom of hyperglycemia.

3. If a client shows symptom of hypoglycemia, they can resume activity once their blood glucose level reaches 100 mg/dL.

4. It is normal for a person's heart to pump at 100 beats per minute or faster.

5. It is probably safe for clients with diabetes to work out at high altitudes.

6. A person with tachycardia may never show symptoms.

7. Strenuous exercise can cause sudden death in non-athletes.

8. Type I diabetes occurs when the body is insulin resistant.

9. Proper instruction and supervision can help prevent injuries.

10. The appropriate response to a diabetic emergency is to:
- a) Call 911 if the person is unconscious.
- b) Give the person fruit juice.
- c) Address any life threatening injuries.
- d) All of the above.

11. True/False: A trainer cannot be sued for negligence if the client signed a consent form.

12. Emergency preparedness includes taking the following steps:
- a) Purchase a fire extinguisher.
- b) Maintain current CPR, AED, and Basic Life Support certifications.
- c) Make sure the client drinks water during the workout.
- d) Have the client sign a waiver.

13. If a client has a seizure, the trainer should:
- a) Lay them on their back.
- b) Go outside and wait for the ambulance.
- c) Restrain the client.
- d) Protect the clients head from injury and place a cushion underneath it.
- e) All of the above.

14. An exercise session should be stopped immediately:
- a) If the client thinks it is too hard.
- b) If the client experiences chest pain.
- c) To make a phone call.
- d) To check the client's pulse.
- e) None of the above.

15. True/False: If a client goes into shock, give them something to drink.

16. A waiver should include the following info:

a) The client's date of birth.
b) The name of the personal training business or club.
c) The client's workout goals.
d) The trainer's phone number.

17. True/False: Elevating a person's legs when they go into shock helps to keep their blood circulating.

18. During a diabetic emergency:

a) Perform CPR.
b) Keep the person warm.
c) Call 911 before doing anything else.
d) None of the above.

19. Musculoskeletal injuries include:

a) Joint dislocations.
b) Bruises.
c) Nose bleeds.
d) Headaches.

20. How much space should be maintained between exercise equipment in a fitness facility?

a) A few inches.
b) 200 feet.
c) 50 feet.
d) 100 feet.

21. True/False: An absolute contraindication to exercise means it is okay to work out under a doctor's supervision.

22. R.I.C.E (rest, ice, compression and elevate) is best administered:

a) 48 hours after the injury occurred.
b) In the morning.
c) At the onset of the injury.
d) When there is bruising.

23. True/False: The cool down should produce the opposite effect of the warm up when done properly.

24. ADA guidelines include which of the following:

a) Doors should be 36 inches wide.
b) If public parking is provided, designated disabled spaces should also be provided.
c) Adequate space for wheelchairs to maneuver inside the facility.
d) All of the above.

25. Define the purpose of the cool down.

a) To get the body ready for exercise.
b) To mimic exercises done during the workout.
c) To transition the body from activity back to a resting state.
d) None of the above.

26. Which is an example of accident prevention?

a) Removing faulty or broken equipment.
b) Encouraging clients to warm up and cool down.
c) Providing towels to clients free of charge.
d) Keep an AED in the fitness facility.

27. True/False: A warm-up should be 2 or 3 minutes in duration.

28. Which is an example of a relative contraindication to exercise testing?

a) Mental impairment leading to an inability to cooperate.
b) Severe hypertension.
c) Inability to speak English.
d) Being deaf.

29. True/False: Clients with osteoporosis should avoid weight training altogether.

30. The three type of stretches are: (circle all that apply)

a) Passive.
b) Aggressive.
c) Active.
d) Ballistic.

31. Stretches should be held for a minimum of:

a) 30 seconds.
b) 1 minute.
c) 2 minutes.
d) As long as you want.

32. Which is a short term effect of exercise?

a) Weight loss.
b) Mobility.
c) Increased Metabolism.
d) All of the above.

Test Your Knowledge: Safety, Injury Prevention, and Emergency Procedures – Answers

1. **False**.

2. **True**.

3. **True**.

4. **False**.

5. **False**.

6. **True**.

7. **True**.

8. **False**.

9. **True**.

10. **d)** All of the above.

11. **False**.

12. **b)** Maintain current CPR, AED, and Basic Life Support certifications.

13. **d)** Protect the client's head from injury and place a cushion underneath it.

14. **b)** The client experiences chest pain.

15. **False**.

16. **b)** The name of the personal training business or club.

17. **True**.

18. **d)** None of the above. In a diabetic emergency, first address any life-threatening emergencies. If the person is conscious, provide fruit juice, non-diet soda, or candy. If the person is conscious, but does not feel better approximately five minutes after taking sugar, call 911 immediately. If the person is unconscious, call 911 immediately.

19. **a)** Joint Dislocations.

20. **d)** 100 feet.

21. **False**.

22. **c)** At the onset of the injury.

23. True.

24. d) All of the above.

25. c) To transition the body from activity back to a resting state.

26. a) Removing faulty or broken equipment.

27. False.

28. a) Mental Impairment leading to an inability to cooperate.

29. False.

30. a) Passive; **c)** Active; and **d)** Ballistic.

31. a) 30 seconds.

32. c) Increased Metabolism.

Chapter 8: Human Behavior

Understanding a person's ability to make permanent lifestyle changes is crucial to health fitness professionals. Your client's attitudes, perspectives, and motivations will influence all of their interactions with you. You cannot simply regurgitate information at your client and expect them to respond – there is much more involved: keeping your clients happy and satisfied; knowing the proper way to instruct your audience; and, above all, making permanent, positive health changes in peoples' lives.

Learning Theories

There are four standard learning theories with human behavior: Behaviorism; Cognitivism; Constructionism; and Humanism.

The first theory, **Behaviorism**, simply views learners as observers who develop, or learn, their behavior based on the type of outside feedback they receive. When people receive positive feedback following an event or action, they learn to repeat the behavior that caused that event or action to occur, while negative feedback prevents reoccurrences.

> For example: Touching a hot stove leads to pain – negative feedback – and so a person learns to never touch the stove again.

The learner is viewed as passive, until acted upon by environmental stimuli (this behavior is also called **operant conditioning**). One way to remember Behaviorism is that people learn through feedback from their *actions*, or how they *behave*.

Cognitivism replaced Behaviorism in the 1960s as the dominant paradigm of learning. Instead of seeing learned behaviors as responses to stimuli, Cognitivism argues that a person's learning process is affected by their own unique thinking, memory, and problem-solving abilities. When dealing with this theory, you'll often see the metaphor of the mind being a computer: information comes in and is processed, leading to certain outcomes.

Constructionism further focuses on the idea that people have unique sequences of learning experiences, and holds that these past experiences affect the way people process new information. Under this theory, learning becomes an active, *constructive* process, where people link new information to prior knowledge in order to build upon their own subjective representations of objective reality.

Humanism, the final and most complex theory, holds that learners must be evaluated entirely in order to understand, interpret, and predict their reactions to new information. Each person's learning is unique and personal to their own self. Combining both affective and cognitive values, this theory emphasizes the potential in every *human*. Humanism learning is student-centered and personal; seeking to ultimately develop confident and self-actualized people in a supportive setting.

After becoming familiar with these learning theories, remember that every person's ability to learn is affected by the type of feedback they receive, in addition to their social background, life experiences, current beliefs and internal disposition. To help clients learn to be fit, professionals must design unique and specific programs accordingly.

Learning Phases

In addition to understanding the four standard learning theories, health fitness professionals can further help clients achieve fitness goals by providing appropriate input during each of three learning phases. These phases occur in the order of:

1. **Cognitive**: Clients focus on learning the basics of a particular exercise or weight machine. Because the activity is new, they must first think about every move before executing it. Full attention will be given to the given instructions and guidance; therefore, health fitness professionals must deliver thorough instructions in order to build the client's confidence levels.

2. **Associative**: This is where muscle memory comes into play. At this point, clients become more comfortable with an exercise and can rely on muscle memory to perform the basic mechanics. They will still depend upon corrections on form or technique, so be prepared to provide constructive criticism at this stage.

3. **Automatic**: Finally, in this phase of learning, clients can perform an exercise efficiently without giving much thought to proper form or technique. Muscle memory will help them automatically make corrections. Positive feedback and further instruction – if necessary – are appropriate in this phase.

What Affects Behavior?

These next theories focus on variables that affect human behavior and explain why people can lack motivation to improve their lives.

The **Health Belief Model** is one such theory that can help identify psychological reasons for a person's inactivity by evaluating their current attitudes and beliefs as a set of variables, depending upon individual perceptions, modifying factors, and the likelihood of action. Note the chart on the following page for how these factors are all related.

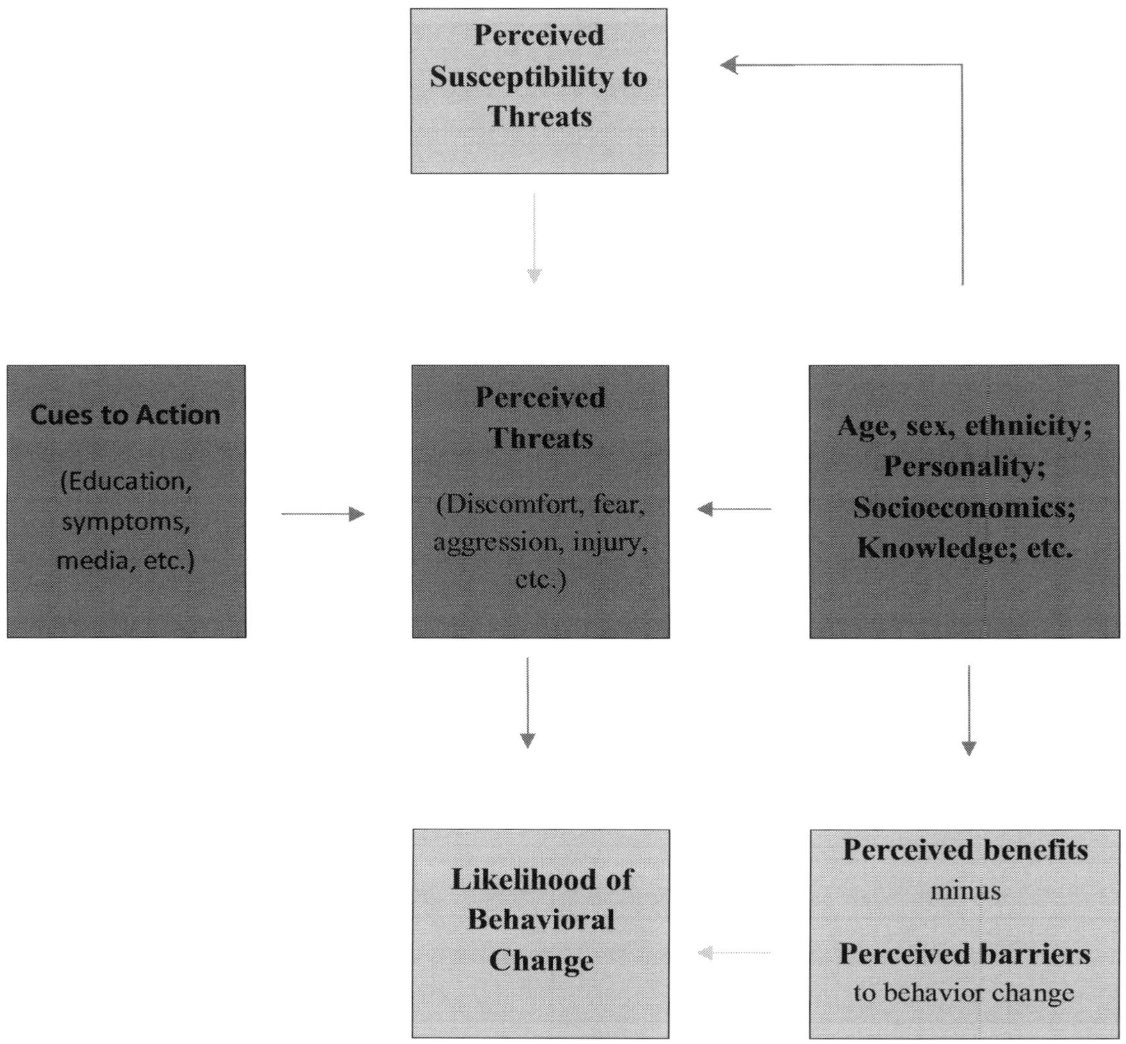

Perceived threats are those fears that exercise will either cause injury or increase a pain that already exists. You must be aware of your clients' fears. Move slowly at first. Never try to push clients to do too much too soon.

Perceived benefits are the benefits of exercise that a client is aware of. These benefits are well-documented, but it is a health fitness professional's responsibility to educate clients about how exercise can directly improve their overall health and any personal fitness challenges they have. People value medical opinions; so, if possible, receive support from the client's physician.

Perceived barriers are the reasons people give for not exercising regularly. Many people feel they don't have the time, funds, or physical abilities to exercise. You must listen to your clients' concerns and work with them to develop ways around any barriers.

Changing Behavior

Behavior change occurs in stages. The **Trans-theoretical Model of Change in Behavior** (TMC) is a model discerning the six stages of change that people go through when developing new patterns of behavior. These stages, listed below, explain how levels of both a willingness to change and motivation vary with progress.

1. **Pre-Contemplation**: The first stage of TMC. In this stage, a person is not open to making lifestyle changes and is possibly in denial of the fact that any modifications are needed. Often, because it is challenging to help clients in this stage change their behavior, various modes of media advertisements are used to help raise exercise awareness.

2. **Contemplation**: The stage wherein which people begin to consider making healthy changes. They haven't taken any steps toward making a change, but they've developed the intention to do so. People in this stage often make resolutions to begin exercising on or right after a certain date, such as the first day of a new year or a milestone birthday.

3. **Preparation**: In the **Preparation** stage, people are actually making an effort to put a fitness plan in motion. They may sign up for a class, join a gym, or purchase athletic gear; but they have not yet adopted new fitness-oriented behaviors.

4. **Action**: The fourth and most critical stage of change, in which people begin activities and programs. Their receiving ongoing encouragement and direction is crucial at this point, because many people become discouraged when changes do not occur as immediately as they had hoped.

   Because of this, the Action stage sees a high rate of drop-out, so health fitness professionals need to be as proactive as possible. Try working with clients to establish specific short term goals in order to show progress. For example: Set measurable goals, like losing a certain number of pounds or increasing the number of repetitions per machine by a specific amount.

   You can even set one-time goals for clients to work on between sessions, such as not snacking after dinner for two days in a row. These goals are more readily attainable, and therefore empowering to your client. Be sure to provide specific verbal praise when clients show improvement (and even point out their progress in areas other than weight loss). Let clients know that you believe in them.

The SMART System of Goal-Setting Can Ensure Success	
Specific	Detail a set desire.
Measurement	Establish a tangible goal.
Action-Oriented	Name the planned steps to success.
Realistic	Keep it doable!
Timed	Establish a realistic time frame.

5. **Maintenance**: The stage in which people have achieved a higher, maintainable level of fitness and adopted a lifestyle that supports continued health. They are now maintaining this healthy behavior.

6. **Termination**: Remains possible even for people who fluctuate between the Action and Maintenance stages. As the name suggests, people in this stage quit, or terminate, the program. To prevent termination, keep clients focused on fitness goals and moving through the stages of change, it is essential for health fitness professionals to use motivational strategies, support, and rewards to match their clients' current positions.

Educate your clients about how using cues can keep them focused. Cues can be anything that reminds a client to stay on the fitness track; for example, post-it note motivational quotes on mirrors.

Processes of Behavioral Change

Within the **Trans-theoretical Model of Change** are ten processes called the Processes of Behavioral Change; five of which are cognitive processes most effective when used during the initial stages of change. The other five are behavioral processes, more useful during the Action and Maintenance stages.

The Five Cognitive Processes:

1. The first cognitive process is **Consciousness Raising**. This can consist of marketing strategies such as special offers for gym memberships, or advertisements about the benefits of good nutrition and the health risks associated with inactivity.

2. **Dramatic Relief** includes using strategies such as psychodrama, grieving losses, and role playing in order to experience and express feelings about a problem preventing exercise.

3. **Environmental Reevaluation** targets specific habits. For example: If targeting smoking, you would provide the client with information about the dangers associated with direct and second-hand smoke.

4. **Self-Reevaluation** occurs when a fitness novice's knowledge and understanding of exercise's benefits increases; at that point, they gain motivation. Health fitness professionals can begin educating new clients about the health gains associated with higher fitness levels during the Preparation stage.

5. **Social Liberation** is the final cognitive process through which people realize that increased health and fitness levels open up opportunities that weren't previously available.

The Five Behavioral Processes:

1. **Counterconditioning** involves the replacement of an unwanted habitual behavior with a healthier alternative. From a fitness standpoint, the unwanted behavior is a habit that keeps someone from achieving improved health.

   For example, a client often forgoes his 5 p.m. workout because he forgets to bring sweatpants to the office. In this scenario, his personal trainer can suggest places to go walking in professional attire. This option keeps the client engaged in something active.

2. **Helping Relationships** promote supportive social bonds, possibly with other health club members, as a means to staying on task with fitness.

3. **Reinforcement Management** provides a reward for good behavior, which reinforces that good behavior. With exercise, the health benefits tend to serve as the reward for people who have already adopted an active lifestyle. However, for clients who are still progressing through the initial stages of change, personal trainers need to use more immediate forms of positive reinforce. For example, offer specific verbal praise when a client shows improvement in form

4. **Self-Liberation** occurs during the final stages of change, when people discover a love for a particular exercise or activity and then make it a permanent part of their routine. It is a personal trainer's duty to help clients discover activities that are enjoyable and rewarding enough to become habits.

5. **Stimulus control** means removing anything that supports the reoccurrence of a bad habit. For instance, giving away the cookie jar if cutting sugar from your diet.

Decisional Balance is another component of The Trans-theoretical Model of Change. This part of the model, from a fitness perspective, looks at how people view the pros and cons of a healthy lifestyle as they move through the stages of change. In the beginning, the cons outweigh the pros, but this balance reverses by the time they reach the final stage (Maintenance).

Self-Efficacy is synonymous with self-confidence. We'll cover it in greater detail on the next page.

Behavioral Strategies to Enhance Physical Activity Participation and Health

Social Cognitive Theory

Social Cognitive Theory identifies and explains the reciprocal interaction of behavioral, personal, and environmental influences and the way this interaction creates unique behavior patterns. The Social Cognitive Theory focuses on the idea of a reciprocal dynamic involving personal, behavioral and environmental influences – in other words, people influence and are influenced by their environments.

SCT Dynamic Model

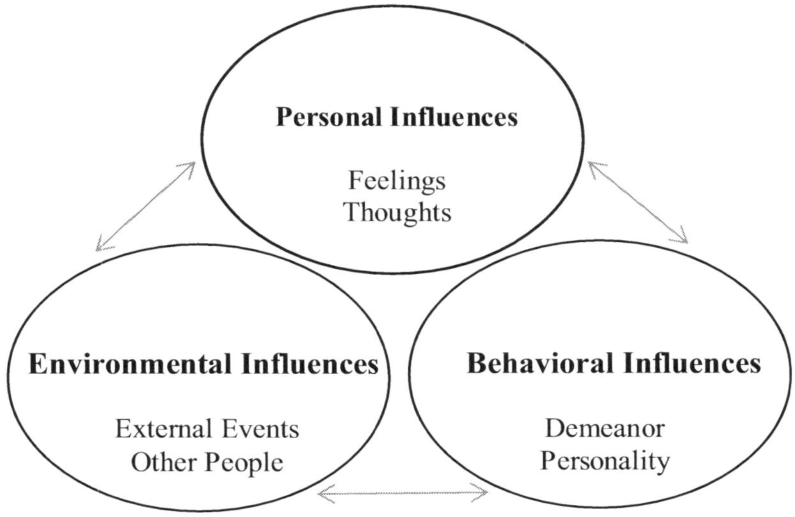

This three-way dynamic reciprocal relationship creates unique realities for every individual, because each part is intrinsically tied to the others. People's thoughts, feelings, beliefs, demeanors, and life experiences all affect the way they view and comprehend events taking place around them.
These events, or environmental influences, are likewise shaped by the actions of the people who are present. For example, a person with a strong personality and a person with a reserved demeanor will most likely have different experiences in similar circumstances. They will evoke different attitudes from the people around them and, as a result, observe different results.

Key Constructs of SCT:

1. Observational Learning.
2. Reinforcement.
3. Self-Efficacy.

When people observe others receiving rewards for certain actions, the observers are likely to partake in the same behavior. For example: A young child sees that her older sister receives praise for clearing her plate. Wanting to receive praise as well, the young child also clears her plate. This is the main thrust of **Observational Learning**, which emphasizes the importance of having positive role models who consistently demonstrate the benefits of fitness.

Likewise, positive **Reinforcement** is essential for someone who is on their way to making exercise a permanent practice. Health fitness professionals can initially be the sole providers of positive reinforcement, so it is important to help clients in the early stages of change to feel good about small accomplishments.

The most important component of SCT from a fitness stand point is **Self-Efficacy**. When a person has self-efficacy, they know they have all the knowledge they need to confidently walk into any health club. Health fitness professionals must equip their clients with the knowledge and support they need to achieve this level of confidence. There are many ways to do this, but some basic ideas can be: informing clients how to adjust seats, change weight loads, and program cardio equipment; letting a client know what to expect when walking into a new environment; or even walking them through the steps they'll be taking in their program to improve confidence.

Another important aspect of helping clients gain self-efficacy is simply acknowledging and addressing their fears and doubts. To do this, effective health fitness professionals must hone their **active listening** skills so their clients feel important, safe, and understood. Active listening means that the focus is completely on the speaker. As active listeners, health fitness professionals must have open body language, make direct eye contact, and ensure that no unnecessary multitasking takes place. Also, it is important for health fitness professionals to not be assuming they already know what clients are about to say or thinking about a response before clients have finished speaking.

Be sure not to interrupt clients while they are speaking, but do use gestures and facial expressions that relay understanding, such as nodding, to show you are actively listening. Lastly, allow a pause at the end of the conversation to make sure clients have finished and then paraphrase back main points for clarification.

Feedback and Reinforcement Methods

Feedback is an important way to let clients know they have your attention. More importantly, specific positive feedback is an effective tool for keeping clients motivated during the initial stages of change.

Extrinsic rewards are tangible items such as free t-shirts or training sessions after clients complete an established goal.

These extrinsic rewards work well in the early stages, but trainers need to help clients realize **intrinsic rewards** for prolonged success. Intrinsic rewards are the benefits that come when clients attain a higher level of fitness. The improved health and wellness at this point serve as the rewards that inspire permanent success.

Test Your Knowledge: Human Behavior

1. Which of the following is synonymous with self-efficacy?
   a) Self-Reevaluation.
   b) Self Confidence.
   c) Self-Liberation.
   d) Self-Control.

2. Why are intrinsic rewards more important than extrinsic rewards?
   a) They provide instant motivation for novice fitness participants.
   b) They provide negative feedback to promote correction.
   c) They are internal rewards that ensure permanent adherence to fitness participation.
   d) They eliminate initial barriers to change.

3. In which of the stages of change is it imperative for personal trainers to be the most proactive?
   a) Contemplation.
   b) Preparation.
   c) Action.
   d) Maintenance.

4. If a person vows to quit smoking on their 30th birthday, which stage of change are they in?
   a) Pre-Contemplation.
   b) Preparation.
   c) Action.
   d) Maintenance.

5. True/False: Getting a free t-shirt with a paid gym membership is an example of an extrinsic reward.

6. In which of the three learning phases would people rely completely on muscle memory to perform an activity?
   a) Cognitive.
   b) Associative.
   c) Automatic.
   d) None of the above.

7. Which of the following is not an example of active listening?
   a) Using open body language.
   b) Forming a response while someone is speaking.
   c) Allowing a pause after a speaker is finished.
   d) Paraphrasing what a speaker has said.

8. True/False: Behaviorism takes into account an individual's past experiences.

9. People may be in denial about the need for behavior modification during the ________ stage of change in the Trans-theoretical Model.

10. Which of the following is an example of a perceived threat according to the Health Belief Model?

a) I can't afford a gym membership.
b) I don't have time to exercise.
c) I already have pain in my knees.
d) Fitness machines are boring.

11. True/False: Personal, behavioral, and environmental influences have little or no effect on each other.

12. True/False: People sometimes fluctuate between the Action and Maintenance stages of change.

13. True/False: Observational learning involves mimicking behavior that appears to be rewarding.

14. Using a workout video when your friend can't meet you at the gym is an example of :

a) Counterconditioning.
b) Self re-evaluation.
c) Stimulus control.
d) Decisional Balance.

15. True/False: The pros outweigh the cons during the final stages of change in the Trans-theoretical Model of Change.

Test Your Knowledge: Human Behavior – Answers

1. **b)** Self Confidence.
2. **c)** They are internal rewards that ensure permanent adherence to fitness participation.
3. **c)** Action.
4. **b)** Preparation.
5. **True**.
6. **c)** Automatic.
7. **b)** Forming a response while someone is speaking.
8. **False**.
9. **Pre-contemplation**.
10. **c)** I already have pain in my knees.
11. **False**.
12. **True**.
13. **True**.
14. **a)** Counterconditioning.
15. **True**.

Chapter 9: Electrocardiography and Diagnostic Techniques

In previous chapters, we've mentioned the necessity of an ECG in exercise testing. Here, we'll go into greater detail.

Electrocardiographs (ECGs) provide basic information about the physiological condition of the myocardium. ECGs record the electrical impulses that stimulate the myocardium to contract. Heart rate, rhythm, impulse conduction route, pathology, and/or disease of the myocardium can be interpreted from an ECG. ECGs are used routinely in diagnostic cardiology, and since abnormalities can frequently be seen in both healthy and diseased individuals, it is critical to be able to identify and interpret the findings.

Diagnostic exercise testing has multiple purposes and applications: diagnostic, prognostic, and therapeutic (especially concerning exercise prescription). You will play an important role in administering various exercise testing protocols and modalities, often combined with imaging studies. A keen understanding of the procedures and anticipated outcomes is necessary for the success of the test and the wellbeing of the patient.

ECG Rhythm Strips and 12-lead ECG Basic Knowledge

The ECG is an electrical representation of the mechanical function of the heart. It displays the route of depolarization of the myocardial cells, and it is normally a systematic and predictable process.

The ECG is inscribed on a **ruled paper strip**, which provides record of cardiac activity and health status of the heart. **Cardiac monitors** and **telemetry** provide the same information. Just like a graph, ECG paper's horizontal axis represents time, and moves from left to right. The graph is measured in millimeters (mm), and the smallest divisions are one mm high and one mm long. A measure of voltage is displayed vertically in mV, showing the height and depth of a wave. Thin black lines are printed every 1 mm (1 small square), and thick black lines every 5 mm (5 small squares). Between two thick black lines are five small squares, each representing .04 seconds, accounting for .2 seconds.

By measuring along the horizontal axis, the duration of any portion of the cardiac cycle can be determined (see image below). ECG machines are calibrated to record **25 mm/second**. A standard 12-lead ECG spans **10 seconds**.

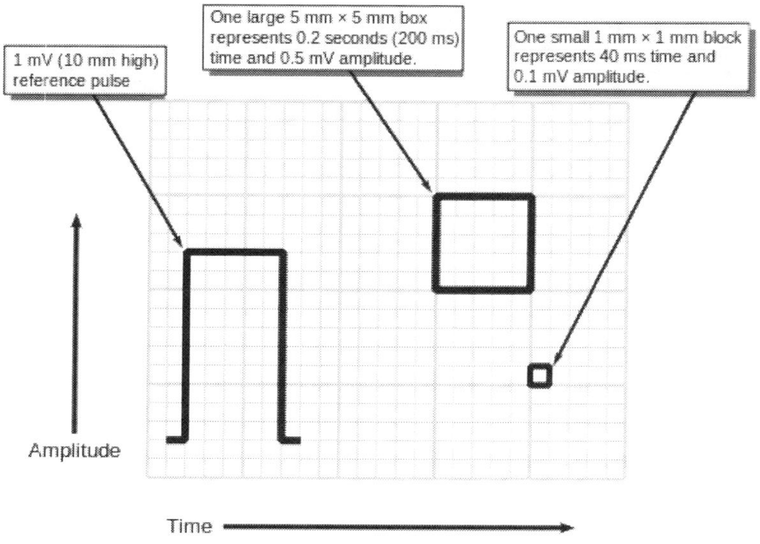

When at rest, the **myocytes**, or muscle cells, have negatively charged (**polarized**) interiors; but, when an electrical stimulus causes them to become positive (a process called **depolarization**), they contract. This depolarization moves as a wave of positive charges through the myocardium (the muscular tissue of the heart). When this wave moves toward a positive skin electrode, it is displayed on the ECG as a **positive deflection**.

Shortly after, the myocytes regain their resting negative charge. This phase is referred to as **repolarization**.

The heart's dominant pacemaker is the **sinus node** (SA Node), located in the upper-posterior wall of the right atrium. The SA Node begins the impulse of depolarization at regular intervals, which spreads outward in a wave fashion, causing the atria to contract. Imagine the atria as a pool of water. A pebble dropped in at the SA Node creates an enlarging, circular wave (depolarization) that spreads outward. This represents the atrial depolarization, which is a spreading wave of positive charges.[i]

When depolarization spreads through both atria, sensitive skin electrodes detect it, and a "**P wave**," a positive deflection, is produced on the ECG. A pause typically follows a P wave, which represents blood passing through the atrioventricular (AV) valves into the ventricles.

Depolarization passes through the **AV node** slowly; but once it reaches the ventricular conduction system, depolarization occurs very quickly through the Bundle of His and the Bundle Branches. Following the stimulus passing through the Bundle of His, Branches, and the Purkinje fibers, depolarization is distributed rapidly to the myocytes of the ventricles. This is represented by what is called the "**QRS complex**" on the ECG.

The QRS complex technically represents the start of ventricular contraction. The **Q wave** (often absent on an ECG) is the first downward stroke of the QRS complex, and is followed by the **R wave**, which is an upward wave.

Remember, if there is any upward deflection in a QRS complex that appears before a Q wave, it is not a Q wave. The upward R wave is followed by a downward **S wave**. This completes the electrical representation of ventricular depolarization.

Following the QRS complex is a segment of horizontal baseline called the "**ST segment**." The ST segment should normally be level with other areas of the baseline. If it is either elevated or depressed beyond normal baseline, it may be indicative of serious pathology. The "**T wave**" follows the ST segment and represents the final rapid phase of ventricular repolarization.

Repolarization occurs so that the ventricular myocytes may recover their resting negative charge within each cell; that way, so they can once again become depolarized. The T wave is usually a low, broad hump. It signifies the end of ventricular systole (contraction), which begins with the Q wave.

To sum it all up, a cardiac cycle is represented by the P wave, the QRS complex, and T wave, and the baseline that follows until another P wave appears.[i]

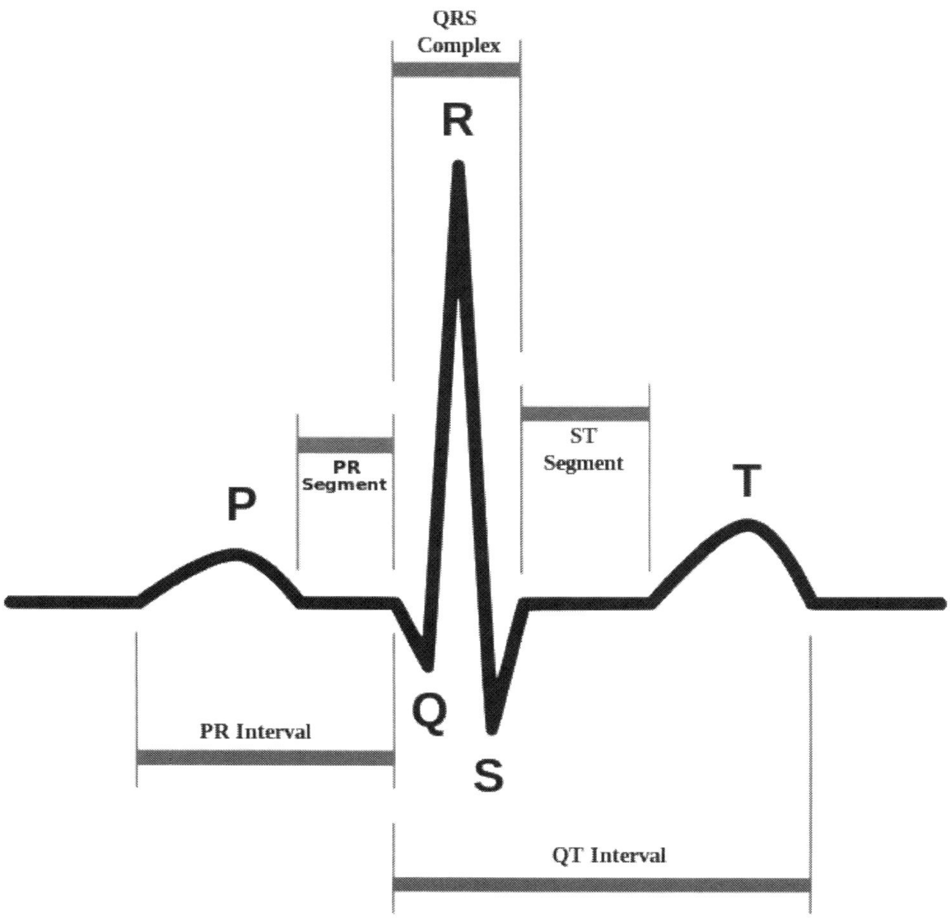

1. P wave: atrial depolarization and contraction
2. QRS Complex: ventricular depolarization and contraction
3. T wave: Ventricular repolarization

The 12-Lead ECG

The standard ECG features 12 **leads**, or pictures of the heart, using 10 wires and electrodes. Electrodes are placed on the chest, wrists, and ankles for a standard 12-lead ECG. This type of ECG is routinely recorded during the **resting phase**, or pre-exercise phase, of an exercise stress test. The combination of these electrodes in different locations provides electrical views of the heart from horizontal, frontal, and vertical planes. Electrodes are placed on both of the arms as well as the left leg to comprise the **limb leads**.

Einthoven's Triangle
Einthoven's Triangle includes leads I, II, and III, where each lead consists of a pair of electrodes. One electrode is positive and one is negative, forming what is called "bipolar" limb leads.

- Lead I views electrical flow from the right arm (negative) to the left arm (positive).
- Lead II views electrical flow from the right arm (negative) to the left leg (positive).
- Lead III views electrical flow from the left arm (negative) to the left leg (positive.)

There are three augmented (meaning amplified) limb leads: aVF, aVR, and aVL.

aVF Lead
The aV**F** lead, which uses the left **F**oot electrode as positive in both right and left arm electrodes, is channeled into a common ground charge with a negative charge. aVF is a cross between leads II and III, hence it being referred to as an "augmented" limb lead. aVR and aVL are obtained similarly.

aVR Lead
For aV**R**, the **R**ight arm electrode is positive, with the remaining two electrodes being negative.

aVL Lead
The aV**L** lead has the **L**eft arm electrode positive, with the other two electrodes being negative. Normally, ECG limb leads will be labeled by color and sometimes labeled according to where they should be placed (i.e., LL for left leg).[i]

There are six chest leads, with positive electrodes placed at six different positions (one per lead). These leads are numbered from V_1 to V_6 and are placed from the patient's right side to their left side. These cover the heart it its anatomical position. All of the chest leads are oriented through the AV node, producing views in a horizontal plane. Imagine leads V_1 through V_6 as spokes of a bicycle wheel. The center of the wheel would be the AV node.

Important Note: While the ECG tracings look slightly different in each lead, remember that the heart's electrical activity does not change from lead to lead, only the angle from which the activity is recorded due to the location of the electrodes.

Leads and Their Corresponding Views of the Heart

I	Lateral	aVR		V_1	Septal	V_4	Anterior
II	Inferior	aVL	Lateral	V_2	Septal	V_5	Lateral
III	Inferior	aVF	Inferior	V_3	Anterior	V_6	Lateral

Skin Preparation Technique

In order to record the most accurate ECG, there are a few steps to take before placing the electrodes to the patient's skin.

1. Have the patient lie in supine position.

2. Locate the correct landmarks for the electrodes.

   Be sure to avoid major muscles, bony protuberances, joints, creases or fatty folds in the skin, areas of skin irritation, and pacemaker sites.

3. If the standard site is not available due to burns, amputation, or another reason, position the landmark site as closely to the standard site as possible.

   In female patients, electrodes are never to be placed on the breast unless access cannot be gained to the normal position. If the electrode is not adhered directly to the skin, **artifact** can be produced, which makes the ECG difficult to interpret. Artifact is defined as ECG abnormalities, which are unrelated to electrical activity of the heart and can distort normal features of the ECG.

   If hair is covering the skin where the electrode is to be placed, the hair should be removed with a disposable razor, which is to be disposed of in a designated sharps container.

4. Next, an alcohol pad is used to clean the skin of any oils or lotions, which hinder adherence of the electrodes.

5. Finally, a piece of sandpaper is used gently on the skin, to help the electrode adhere well. This is especially important when an exercise test is being performed, as movement and sweat could threaten the integrity of the placement.

After these steps have been completed, you can place the electrodes. Attach lead wires to each corresponding electrode, and advise the patient to refrain from moving or speaking while you wait for the 12-lead ECG to appear on the monitor. Be sure to review the quality of the ECG. If artifact is present, correct the cause and obtain another 12-lead ECG.

Trouble-Shooting While Monitoring

ECG signals can be interrupted by various sources. Being aware of these potential interferences will enable you to quickly identify the problem and correct it, producing an accurate ECG recording.

Power Line Interference: Filters within an ECG machine affect power line interference. In a non-adaptive machine, an internally designed filter that is turned at 60Hz removes this interference. An adaptive machine has a built-in adaptable filtering capability for other types of artifact.

Muscle Contraction: Tense muscles in the arm or legs can produce artifact. Encourage your patient to relax in the supine position with limbs supported during ECG recordings.

Faulty Equipment: Loose, dry, or outdated electrodes; a loose lead wire; poor cable connection; or insufficient skin preparation can also mimic artifact. To avoid, keep electrodes in an unopened package until the time of use, and use them before the expiration date. Secure cable connections and check for observable damage to any of the equipment.

Wandering Baseline: Artifacts can be observed during deep inhalations and exhalations, during increased body movement, or when an electrode loses contact with the skin. This type of artifact looks like the baseline is wandering – slowly sloping upward or downward.

Electromagnetic Interference: This type of artifact originates outside of the patient and is caused by interference from electronic sources, such as power cords, AC-powered equipment that may be insufficiently grounded, and/or nearby use of a hand-held radio.

Standard Chest Lead Placement

Correct electrode placement is very important to be able to determine normal and abnormal function of the myocardium. Precise placement also helps to prevent artifact. The following charts describe the correct locations for the chest and limb leads.

V_1	On right sternal border, in 4th intercostal space.
V_2	On left sternal border, in 4th intercostal space.
V_3	At midpoint on a straight line between V_2 and V_4.
V_4	At the midclavicular line, on 5th intercostal space.
V_5	On the anterior axillary line, horizontal to V_4.
V_6	On the midaxillary line, horizontal to V_4 and V_5.

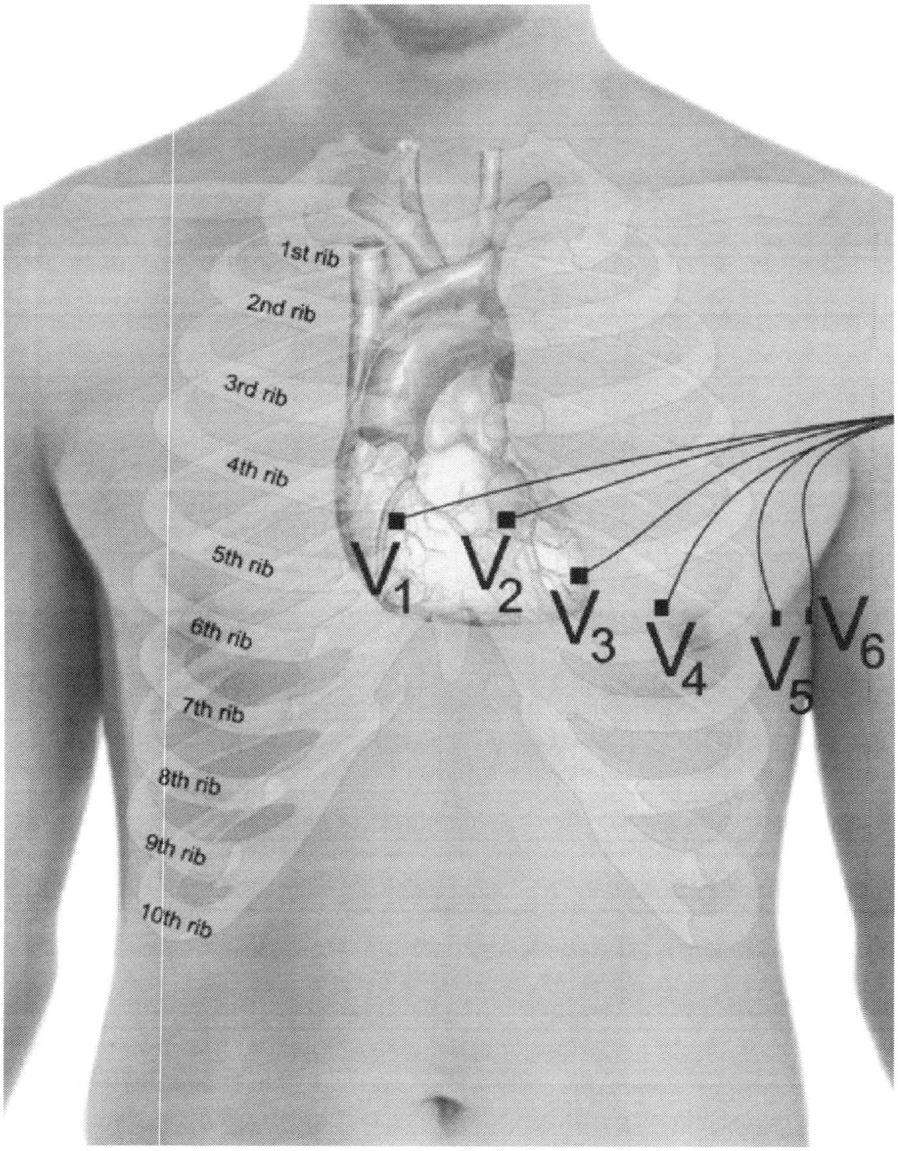

Tip: To find the 4th intercostal space, locate the sternoclavicular joint and place your index finger in the space directly below the first rib. That's the first intercostal space. Continue down the sternum until you locate the 4th space.

Standard Limb Lead Placement

RA (right arm)	White
RL (right leg)	Green
LA (left arm)	Black
LL (left leg)	Red

Tip: To help remember the lead placement, think "white to the right," "clouds over grass," (white above green) and "smoke over fire" (black above red).

Mason Likar Lead System

Limb lead placement is modified for exercise testing by placing the RA and LA electrodes in the subclavian areas (avoiding bone and muscle), and the LA and LL electrodes in the suprailiac areas. This is for safety purposes, preventing any tripping or interference.

Single Lead System

By using either 3 or 5 leads, one can obtain a one-dimensional look at the heart, featuring only heart rate and rhythm. The **5-lead system** is more commonly used, and it features the RA, LA, LL, RL, and V_1 electrodes. The **3-lead system** features only the RA, LA, and LL electrodes. For both methods, electrodes have modified positioning on the torso. RA and LA are placed in the subclavian area, RL and LL are placed in the suprailiac areas, and V_1 is placed in the normal position, on the right of the sternal border, in the 4th intercostal space.

CM5 System

The CM5 lead is useful for the detection of **myocardial ischemia**. Remember that myocardial ischemia occurs when there is a partial or complete blockage in one or more coronary artery, which decreases blood flow, and thus oxygen supply in the heart.

The CM5 lead has the right arm electrode placed on the manubrium of the sternum, and the left arm electrode is placed at the V_5 position (on the anterior axillary line, horizontal to V_4). The left leg lead acts neutrally and may be placed anywhere. The "C" in CM5 stands for clavicle, where it is often placed. This position allows detection of up to 80% of left ventricular ischemia, as well as arrhythmias.

ECG Interpretation and Analysis

Heart Rate

Heart rate can be defined as the number of electrical impulses conducted through the myocardium in one minute. Each area of the heart has an inherent heart rate.

The **atrial rate** is determined by the number of P waves seen.

The **ventricular rate** is determined by the number of R waves seen.

The SA node is the pacemaker of the heart, and the heart rate should be between 60-100 beats per minute (bpm). If the SA node fails to fire, there are other potential pacemakers in the heart, which can fire, a process referred to as "**automaticity foci**."

However, if the impulse originates from somewhere other than the SA node, and that impulse fires faster than the SA node, it can temporarily or permanently take over, and this is evidenced by ectopic/premature beats.[i] This is referred to as "**irritability**."

Tip: Heart rate represents electrical activity. Pulse represents perfusion to the target tissues. Heart rate is not always the same as the pulse! **Treat the patient, not the monitor!**

Normal Heart Rates: Inherent Rates

SA Node (Sinus Rhythms)	60 – 100 bpm
Atria (Atrial Rhythms)	60 – 80 bpm
AV Node/Junction (Junctional Rhythms)	40 – 60 bpm
Ventricles (Ventricular Rhythms)	20 – 40 bpm

There are four different methods of determining heart rate from a rhythm strip.

1. The first method is to use **division**. Count the number of small squares between two R waves and divide the total number into 1500.

   This is the most accurate, but also the most time-consuming method. Calipers and calculators may be used. The calculation behind this method is 60 seconds * 25 mm/sec = 1500 mm.

2. The next method is a faster one. This is the **countdown method**, where you start with an R wave that peaks on a heavy black vertical line.

   - One large square represents 300 bpm.
   - Two represent 150 bpm.
   - Three represent 100 bpm.
   - Four represent 75 bpm.
   - Five represent 60 bpm.
   - Six represent 50 bpm.

   When using this method, count down until you arrive to the next R wave.

3. Next, a **heart rate ruler** can be used. This is the easiest method. You simply line up the ruler on the horizontal axis and use it to measure heart rate.

4. The final method, the **six-second count**, is used for irregular rhythms. Using a six-second rhythm strip, count the number of R waves, and then multiply that number by ten to estimate the heart rate. This is not a very accurate method, but it works best for irregular rhythms.[i]

When a normal sinus rhythm has a rate less than 60 bpm, it is classified as "**sinus bradycardia**." This rhythm originates in the SA node, and features the characteristics of a normal rhythm, only slowed.

When a normal sinus rhythm has a rate greater than 100 bpm, it is classified as "**sinus tachycardia**." This rhythm also originates in the SA node and features the characteristics of a normal rhythm, only more rapid.

Note that as the heart beats faster, the QRS complexes get closer together, and P waves may be "lost."

The Cardiac Cycle
Each feature of the cardiac cycle on the ECG has a set of normal characteristics, indicating healthy heart tissue. It's integral to know these features well, so that abnormalities and irregularities can be identified. Look at the following chart, and learn the characteristics listed.

***Remember, in the QRS complex, the Q wave is the first negative deflection, the R wave is the first positive deflection, and the S wave is the second negative deflection.

	P Wave	**PR Interval**	**QRS Complex**	**T Wave**	**QT Interval**
Normal Measures	• < .12 sec width. • < 3 mm amplitude.	• .12 – .20 seconds. • < .12 sec = Junctional. • > .20 sec = AV Blocks.	• < .12 seconds.	• Amplitude is < 10 mm in chest leads.	• < .40 seconds.
Normal Appearance	Positive and rounded in leads I, II, AVF, $V_4 - V_6$. Positive, negative, or biphasic in leads III, AVL, $V_1 - V_3$.	Measured from the beginning of P wave to beginning of QRS complex.	Amplitude varies from lead to lead and person to person. Dependant on size of ventricular chambers and proximity of chest electrodes to ventricular chamber.	Usually round and upright in leads I, II, and V_2-V_6. Inverted in AVR. Inverted/biphasic in V1, II.	Measured from beginning of QRS complex to end of T wave. Should be less than half the R-R interval.

Important Note: Under the "QRS Comlex" column, ventricular chamber size impacts the amplitude of the complex. The larger the chamber, the larger the complex. A person's weight can affect the complex size as well, because the more overweight a person is, the further the proximity of the chest electrodes to the ventricular chamber, thus the smaller the complex.

Arrhythmias

Arrhythmia literally means "without rhythm," but the term is used to signify any rhythm disturbance – any variance from a normal sinus rhythm. The term "**dysrhythmia**" is used in the same way. Arrhythmias can be divided into several general categories based on the mechanism of origin of the arrhythmia. With any rhythm, patient assessment is essential to determine tolerance of the rhythm or arrhythmia.

Remember the signs of poor cardiac output: pale, cool, clammy skin; cyanosis, dyspnea, confusion, disorientation, dizziness, weakness, fatigue, faintness/syncope; sudden change in blood pressure; nausea, vomiting, decreased urinary output, and loss of consciousness.

Each arrhythmia has its own set of clues or rules. Since there is a wide range of normal variability, it is best to take a systematic approach to identifying them. The systematic approach to identifying rhythms features three steps. Step one is to determine if the **rhythm** is regular or irregular. Step two is to determine the **heart rate**, and step three is to analyze **complex formation**.

To identify whether a heart rhythm is regular or irregular, measure more than two cardiac cycles. Measure R-R intervals for ventricular regularity, and measure P-P intervals for atrial regularity. If there is < .06 of a second of variability, an interval can be deemed as regular. A > .06 second of variability signifies an irregularity. If a rhythm is irregular, ask yourself if there is a pattern to the irregularity. Is the rhythm regularly irregular (a pattern of irregularity)? Is the rhythm basically irregular (a regular rhythm with a beat or two interrupting it)? Or is the rhythm totally irregular, with no patterns at all?

Next, determine the exact heart rate. If the rhythm is irregular, use the six-second count. Compare the atrial and ventricular heart rates. Remember that the number of P waves seen determines the atrial rate, and the number of R waves seen determines the ventricular rate. Are the two rates the same?

Concerning complex formation, examine each cardiac cycle from the beginning to end. Starting with the P waves, here are some questions to ask: are P waves present? Are they all upright? Do they all look alike? Is there a P wave before every QRS complex? Are the P-P intervals equal? To help determine if a wave is a P wave, set calipers at .20 seconds in front of the QRS complex. If a wave is there, it is likely to be a P wave. P waves are the most reliable of all waves.

Next, look at the PR intervals. Ask yourself, are they all present? Are they equal? Are all PR intervals within a normal range of .12 – .20 seconds?

Look at the QRS complex next. Are all QRS complexes present? Do all of the complexes look alike? Is there a QRS complex after every P' wave? Are the R-R intervals equal and within the normal ranges of < .12 seconds?

Learning to ask yourself these questions when interpreting an ECG is a good habit. It makes identifying arrhythmias less confusing, and more systematic.

Types of Arrhythmias

There are many types of arrhythmias you may come across, and while it is beneficial to be able to recognize all of them, only the most prevalent arrhythmias will be discussed below.

Atrial Fibrillation

This common irregular rhythm, often called "A-fib," is caused by the continuous, rapid-firing of multiple atrial automaticity foci. No single impulse depolarizes the atrial completely, and only an occasional atrial depolarization gets through the AV node to stimulate the ventricles. This produces an irregular ventricular (QRS) rhythm. There are no true P waves in A-fib, due to no single impulse completely depolarizing, so there are only a rapid series of tiny, erratic spikes on the ECG. There is an irregular ventricular response, and it may result in either a slow or rapid ventricular rate, however, it is always irregular.[i] This is an important arrhythmia to know, because it increases risk for developing atrial thrombus, which may lead to stroke or other embolic events.

Ventricular Fibrillation (V-Fib)

V-Fib is a type of **cardiac arrest**, because there is no pumping action by the heart. It requires immediate CPR and defibrillation. It is caused by rapid-rate discharges from many extremely irritable ventricular automaticity foci, producing an erratic, rapid twitching of the ventricles, with a ventricular rate of 350 – 450 bpm. This erratic twitching of V-Fib is referred to as "a bag of worms," due to its appearance, with no identifiable waves, and the ventricles do not provide mechanical pumping. Note: If you recognize any repetition of pattern or regularity of deflections, you are probably not dealing with V-Fib.

Atrial Flutter

Atrial flutter occurs when an extremely irritable atrial automaticity focus fires at a rate of 250 – 350 per minute, producing a rapid series of atrial depolarizations. Atrial flutter is easily identified by a series of identical "flutter" waves in rapid back-to-back succession, which resemble the appearance of the teeth of a saw.

Multifocal Atrial Tachycardia (MAT)

Since three or more atrial foci are involved in this arrhythmia, P waves appear in various shapes. Due to the multifocal origin of MAT, each individual atrial focus paces at its own inherent rate, but the total, combined "normal" pacing of multiple unsuppressed foci produces a rapid, irregular rhythm. In a given lead, each focus produces P waves with a specific morphology. MAT is also sometimes associated with **digitalis toxicity** in patients with heart disease.[i]

Paroxysmal Junctional Tachycardia

The sudden rapid pacing of a very irritable automaticity focus in the AV Junction causes this arrhythmia. The term "paroxysmal" refers to the spastic nature of the automaticity focus. The Junctional focus may suddenly initiate tachycardia pacing because of marked irritability, induced by stimulants and/or a premature heart beat from another focus. This arrhythmia paces at the rate of 150 – 250 bpm.

Note that a rapidly pacing, or irritable, Junctional focus *may* also depolarize the atria from below in a retrograde, or backwards way, to produce an inverted P immediately before each QRS Complex; or an inverted P after each QRS Complex; or an inverted P buried within each QRS, which is difficult to identify.[i]

Premature Atrial Complexes (PACs)
Premature atrial complexes (PACs) and premature ventricular complexes (PVCs) are not life-threatening, and they occur often during exercise or other periods when catecholamine levels are elevated. PACs occur when an atrial site other than the sinus node depolarizes prematurely. The impulse proceeds through the AV node and the ventricles to produce a narrow QRS complex. When a series of normal beats alternate with PACs, it is called "**atrial bigeminy**." When a PAC occurs every third beat, it's called "**trigeminy**," and every fourth is called "**quadrigeminy**".[ii]

Premature Ventricular Complexes (PVCs)
PVCs occur when a site in the ventricles fires before the next wave, or when depolarization from the sinus node reaches the ventricle. P waves are often not present, or are hidden, and PVCs usually feature wide QRS complexes; they may occur alone, in pairs (couplet), groups (triplet), or in runs.

With multiform PVCs, the PVC waveform changes from beat to beat, signifying that the PVC may come from more than one foci in the ventricle; or it may be the product of more than one physiologic process. PVCs occur prematurely, and are followed by a compensatory pause.[ii] Remember to identify the underlying rhythm when PVCs or PACs are present.

Ventricular Tachycardia (V Tach)
V Tach is produced by a very irritable ventricular automaticity focus that suddenly paces in the 150 – 250 bpm range. It features a characteristic pattern of huge, consecutive PVC-like complexes. During V Tach, the SA Node continues to pace the atria, but only a sporadic atrial depolarization catches the AV Node in a responsive state; and then this depolarization stimulus conducts to the ventricles.

Runs of V Tach may signify coronary ischemia or other causes of **cardiac hypoxia** (lack of oxygen), which makes a ventricular automaticity focus very irritable. Note that this rapid rate is too fast for the heart to effectively function, especially in those elderly individuals with compromised coronary arteries. That is why this is an important arrhythmia to recognize and treat quickly in patients with a heart attack.

Supraventricular Tachycardia (SVT)
SVT is any arrhythmia that is initiated above the AV node. SVT describes a category, not just one rhythm. Both atrial fibrillation and flutter fit into this category. SVT can be thought of as "narrow QRS tachycardia," due to its appearance. SVT originates from an irritable site above the bundle of His.

Important Note: When interpreting an arrhythmia, to determine if it is supraventricular or ventricular, look at the width of the QRS complex. Know that the wider the complex, the more likely that the beat is ventricular. Remember that ventricular rhythms are life threatening!

Asystole
When there is no electrical activity at all, the patient is considered to be in asystole. There are no waveforms, just a straight or wavy line. At this point defibrillation no longer is initiated.

Diagnostic Stress Testing

Indications
There are several indications for conducting clinical stress tests. These tests are an extension of the patient's medical history and physical examination (covered in-depth in the previous chapters), which allow the physician to examine the patient in circumstances that will provoke the signs or symptoms of cardiovascular or pulmonary disease. Stress tests evaluate exertional discomfort, including chest

discomfort, dyspnea, leg discomfort, palpitations, and neurological symptoms. Stress tests also evaluate the presence of occult coronary artery disease and provide information regarding risk stratification in those with known cardiovascular disease. Testing can also aid in prescribing exercise and follow-up therapy. In summary, performing a stress test serves diagnostic purposes, allows for functional evaluation, and determines prognosis or risk.[ii]

Contraindications

For some, the risks of exercise testing outweigh the potential benefits. For these patients, it's imperative to cautiously examine risk versus benefit when making the decision to perform an exercise test. To help identify potential contraindications, it is wise to perform a pre-exercise test evaluation, as well as a careful review of the patient's medical history. Patients with absolute contraindications should not perform exercise tests until such conditions are stabilized or appropriately treated. Those with relative contraindications may be tested after careful evaluation of the risk/benefit ratio.

A comprehensive list of the absolute and relative contraindications to exercise testing can be found in the *ACSM Guidelines for Exercise Testing and Prescription 8th ed., Box 3.5* (GETP8 Box 3.5).

An absolute contraindication is a recent significant change in the resting ECG that suggests significant ischemia, recent myocardial infarction (within 2 days), or other acute cardiac events. Unstable angina, uncontrolled symptomatic cardiac dysrhythmias, and symptomatic severe aortic stenosis are also on the list of *absolute* contraindications. Left main coronary stenosis, moderate stenotic valvular heart disease, and electrolyte abnormalities are among the list of *relative* contraindications.

It's important to know that contraindications may not apply in several specific clinical situations, including: soon after acute myocardial infarction; revascularization procedure; or bypass surgery to determine the need for, or benefit of, drug therapy.

Also, there are some conditions that preclude dependable diagnostic ECG information from stress testing, such as a left bundle-branch block or digitalis therapy. In these circumstances, the exercise test may still provide beneficial information regarding exercise capacity, dysrhythmias, and hemodynamic responses to exercise. Additional evaluative techniques including respiratory gas exchange analyses, echocardiography, or nuclear imaging can be combined with the exercise test to improve sensitivity, specificity, and diagnostic capabilities.[iii]

Procedures

Just as with the exercise testing covered in previous chapters, you must – before beginning a stress test – present an informed consent document and review it with the patient before obtaining a signature, due to a certain risk of complications during the test. It's very important to explain to the patient what they are likely to experience and feel during the test and that the purpose is to elicit the signs and symptoms of cardiovascular or pulmonary disease.

Next, it is wise to review the patient's history, current medications, and indications for the test, along with any current or recent changes in symptoms, to confirm that the goals of the test are well understood by everyone involved in the testing.

Lastly, the resting ECG should be recorded and examined before starting the test. It's important to identify any contraindications for testing and ensure that the resting ECG is adequately normal to allow for interpretation of changes that may occur during the exercise test. If there are more than the minimal abnormalities on the resting ECG, adjunctive procedures should be considered if the purpose of the test is to make a new diagnosis.

Usually these adjunctive procedures would include radionuclide myocardial perfusion imaging and either radionuclide or echocardiographic measurements of left ventricular function. Additional imaging tests are not required when the goal of the test is to determine functional capacity.

The next procedure is to choose the appropriate exercise mode. The treadmill exercise test is the most-commonly performed in the United States. For those who are unable to use a treadmill due to being overweight or having lower-limb limitations, other modes are appropriate, such as arm ergometry or seated stepping.

Next, be sure that the appropriate personnel are present. For exercise stress testing of patients with high-risk medical conditions (heart failure or high-grade dysrhythmias), it is suggested to have direct physician supervision. For other cases, having a supervising physician who is readily available to respond to questionable interpretations or emergencies in the immediate area is appropriate.[ii]

Protocols

Exercise testing protocols provide an appropriate method for conducting the test for the professional and the patient. While there are many types of testing protocols, using both cycle ergometry and treadmills, the Bruce treadmill protocol is the most widely used protocol in the United States. For those who are older and weaker, the high starting aerobic demand and large increases in speed and grade (incline) between stages requires another protocol to be considered. The modified Bruce treadmill tests are popular for this population. Refer to GETP8 Figure 5-3 to familiarize yourself with other popular protocols.

Before, throughout, and after the test, heart rate, blood pressure, and perceived exertion using the Borg scale (RPE scale) should be monitored and documented. ECG monitoring should occur continuously, including during resting, with the patient in supine and exercise position. Remember, it is normal for heart rate to increase with increasing workloads. Both blood pressure and RPE should be assessed in the final 30 – 60 seconds of each stage of the test, and again at peak exercise and through the recovery stage, for at least 6 – 8 minutes to ensure a normal cool-down.

When measuring blood pressure while the patient is exercising, it is often easier to have the patient rest one arm on your shoulder, instead of while gripping a treadmill handrail. A tight grip on the treadmill can produce noise interference that can prevent hearing auscultation sounds, and can make accurate measurements difficult. Throughout the test, the ECG should be monitored for any ST-segment abnormalities (indicating ischemia or injury, to be discussed later) or arrhythmias.

Assess standard chest pain evaluations and, if appropriate, evaluate for dyspnea and claudication pain at the end of each stage. If these symptoms are present, then asses more than once per stage.[ii] GETP8 Table 5.2 provides a helpful chart concerning recommended monitoring intervals throughout the test. **Be sure to know these well!**

To decide when to terminate the exercise test, you will find a comprehensive list of absolute and relative indications in GETP8 Box 5-2. We will reiterate several of those absolute indications here:

1. Patient demonstrates a drop in systolic blood pressure of > 10 mm Hg from the baseline blood pressure, despite an increase in workload – accompanied by other signs of ischemia.
2. Patient experiences moderately severe angina (chest pain), defined as 3 on the standard scale.
3. Patient experiences increasing nervous system symptoms, such as ataxia, dizziness, or near syncope.
4. Any sign of poor cardiac perfusion, such as cyanosis or pallor, is another reason to absolutely terminate the test, out of concern for the safety of the patient.

In general, the test should be continued until the question behind the test's initiation has been answered. You should aim to bring the patient to either a fatigue or symptom/sign limitation, to ensure that the information regarding exercise capacity has been acquired.

However, if the patient has demonstrated clear abnormal findings and they have been documented, it is not necessary to continue the test. Some professionals aim to attain 85% of the age-predicted maximal heart rate, believing it is adequate stress for revealing exertional ischemia. However, the sensitivity of exercise testing is increased in tests where more than 85% of the age-predicted heart rate is achieved.

Therefore it's reasonable to argue that achievement of a particular heart rate is more of a security measure in a normal exercise test. While it can be argued that the safest place to provoke abnormal physiological findings is in the exercise laboratory, where complications can be quickly identified and addressed, the risk of acute myocardial infarction (heart attack) is increased when a previously sedentary person performs intense exercise.[ii]

After the stress test, it is best to perform a short period of low-intensity exercise (such as slow walking at no incline), to document the recovery pattern of the patient's heart rate and blood pressure.

This also supports venous return and hemodynamic stability during recovery to prevent hypotension, which can cause significant exertional ischemia by decreasing perfusion pressure into the myocardium. When the patient is cooling down, it is a perfect opportunity to communicate the value of regular exercise, weight loss, smoking cessation, or the safety of resuming activities that the patient may be hesitant about.

Interpreting Results

Remember, exercise testing is usually quite safe. Recent data suggests that the risk of serious complications is less than two out of 10,000 tests. Proper consideration to contraindications for exercise testing, attentive monitoring throughout the test, and recognizing criteria for ending the exercise test all contribute to the safety of the patient.

When interpreting the results of the exercise test, keep in mind at least five factors: clinical responses, ECG responses, exercise capacity, hemodynamic responses, and what the exercise test score says about the patient.

Concerning evidence of symptoms during the test, such as chest discomfort, the timing and character of the chest discomfort must be carefully considered. Also, recognize that in older patients, dyspnea is often an angina equivalent. Ideally, the presence of symptoms will correlate with either ECG or hemodynamic abnormalities. However, know that these can be hidden by baseline ECG abnormalities, arrhythmias, pacemaker activity, or medications.

ST-segment changes on the ECG are classic signs of exertional ischemia. ST-segment depression that is horizontal or down-sloping and > 1mm from the baseline is the minimal diagnostic threshold to support a diagnosis of exertional myocardial ischemia.

ST-segment changes that present early on in the test, are observed in multiple leads, or persist into recovery are predictive either of severe single-vessel cardiovascular disease (CVD) or multivessel disease.

Dysrhythmias, particularly ventricular dysrhythmias, during exercise testing are a cause for concern, because they are presumed to foreshadow major hemodynamic collapse. Usually, when you see dysrhythmias that increase in frequency or complexity with advanced exercise, it is indicative of ischemia or hemodynamic instability, and thought to be more serious than isolated dysrhythmias.

Although most exercise testing is done without direct measurements of respiratory gas exchange, such measurements have proved to be clinically significant. This measurement is the most accurate method of determining functional capacity. A high maximal oxygen uptake (VO_{2max}) can be correlated with a relatively high cardiac output, and therefore the absence of any serious limitations or impairments of left ventricular function. To understand one's exercise capacity, age and sex-predicted norms are used, featuring simple percentages.

It is important to examine **hemodynamic responses** in a diagnostic stress test, because they are used to identify high-risk situations. Abnormalities concerning either the pattern or magnitude of the systolic blood pressure response have historically been recognized as being significant regarding prognosis. A decline in systolic blood pressure, especially when below the pre-exercise level or combined with ECG abnormalities, is widely accepted as a sign of decreasing cardiac output. This is why it has become an absolute point of test termination.

Remember that normal systolic blood pressure increases in a negatively-accelerated manner during incremental exercise. The scale of the normal increase is approximately 10 mm Hg per MET (metabolic equivalent), with a minimal increase of 10 mm Hg from rest to maximal exercise.

An absolute peak systolic pressure greater than 250 mm Hg, or a relative increase greater than 140 mm Hg above resting levels, is considered a hypertensive response and indicates future resting hypertension.

Following the exercise test, systolic blood pressure normally decreases quickly. When this response is delayed, it is highly related to both ischemic abnormalities and a poor prognosis. As a rule-of-thumb, the 3-minute post-exercise systolic blood pressure should be less than 90% of the systolic blood pressure at peak exercise.

Chronotropic incompetence, when a patient cannot achieve an adequate heart rate response to exercise, is a cause for concern during exercise testing. Chronotropic incompetence is linked with a poor prognosis beyond that accounted for by symptoms or ECG abnormalities.

Failure to reach 80% of the predicted heart rate reserve (in those with no pharmacologic reason) is the most widely accepted cut point for diagnosing someone as having a heart rate response limitation. There is great prognostic value of a poor heart rate response indicating an exercise-induced myocardial perfusion deficit.

It is important to note that an abnormal chronotropic response offers information that is independent of myocardial perfusion; the combination of perfusion deficit with an abnormal chronotropic index indicates a worse prognosis than either abnormality by itself. Similarly, the inability of the heart rate to recover quickly after exercise provides independent information related to prognosis. This is related to the inability to reestablish vagal control over heart rate, which is independently known to predispose to arrhythmic heart conditions.[ii]

Radionuclide Testing

In patients with abnormal resting ECGs, exercise testing may be combined with various testing techniques. These techniques can augment the ECG or replace it when resting abnormalities make evaluation of changes during exercise not possible. Different radioisotopes can be used to evaluate the presence of perfusion during exertional ischemia, or to identify abnormalities of ventricular function that often accompany heart attacks or exertional ischemia.

Myocardial perfusion imaging can be done with a variety of agents and imaging approaches, with the most common isotopes being Thallium or Technetium (Cardiolyte). When there has been a myocardial infarction, the necrotic (dead) tissue does not result in uptake of the isotope, so a nonreversible reduction of tracer activity is observed on the image.

In the case of exertional ischemia, the tissue uptake in the affected region is reduced during exercise because of a reduction of blood flow (and thus isotope) to the ischemic tissue during exercise.

Technetium can also be used to evaluate ventricular function, using an ECG gated blood pool. This involves the isotope tagging red cells and recording images over 60 – 120 seconds, producing movies of the brightest spot in the heart while it changes volume throughout the cardiac cycle. This allows for evaluation of the contraction pattern of different walls of the heart. Since ischemic muscle (scar tissue) doesn't contract well, the motion of the wall will decrease throughout an exercise test when the patient reaches a point of exertional ischemia. Myocardial perfusion and ventricular function studies with pharmacologic stress are also used in patients who are incapable of exercising.[ii]

Echocardiographic Imaging

Ultrasound can be utilized to image the heart in relation to exercise or pharmacologic stress. While echocardiographs are not utilized for evaluating myocardial perfusion, it is relatively simple to examine the heart before and after a conventional exercise test. A set of resting images are recorded before the test, and then the exercise test is performed following a normal treadmill protocol, but instead of an extended cool-down, the patient undergoes a second echocardiograph immediately after terminating the exercise portion of the test. This allows for the regional wall motion of various segments of the left ventricle to be recorded. Deterioration in regional wall motion with exercise is indicative of myocardial ischemia.[ii]

Pathologies

Atrioventricular (AV) Blocks

AV Blocks occur when there is a delay within the AV Node, which delays the impulse from the atria, making an abnormally long pause before ventricular contraction. There are four classifications of AV blocks: one of first-degree, two types of second-degree, and one third-degree (or complete) heart block. Heart disease, aging, and pericarditis can cause AV blocks.

- **First-degree AV Block**: This delay features a prolonged PR interval of *more* than one large square (.2 sec) on the ECG. This occurs when the cardiac cycle is consistently normal, but the PR interval is prolonged the same amount in every cycle. This is only a partial block.

- **Second-degree AV Block** (Also called **Wenchebach Block**): This occurs when the PR interval becomes progressively longer from cycle to cycle, until the AV Node will no longer conduct a stimulus from above. You will see the PR interval gradually become longer until a QRS complex is *"dropped."* You will see that the whole rhythm is irregular, and that there are more P waves than QRS complexes.

- **Second-degree AV Block (Mobitz)**: This occurs when a normal, *punctual P wave is not followed by a QRS response*; and the other cycles usually have normal PR intervals. There is no progressive lengthening of the PR-interval in a Mobitz. A Mobitz will never feature a premature P wave, so be aware of that.

- **Third-degree AV Block**: This is a complete AV block, where none of the atrial depolarizations conduct to the ventricles. When this happens, an automaticity focus below the block escapes overdrive suppression to pace the ventricles at its inherent rate.

You will find normal, narrow QRS complexes, with a ventricular rate of 40 – 60 bpm if there is a junctional focus. If there is a ventricular focus, you will find PVC-like QRS complexes and a ventricular rate of 20 – 40 bpm. Know that in complete AV block, the ventricular rate may be so slow that there is insufficient blood flow to the brain, causing syncope in the patient.[i]

To help with identifying blocks, consider the following:

- If there is a missed P-QRS-T cycle, there is a sinus block.

- A punctual P wave, with no QRS response, indicates an AV conduction block (Mobitz).

- A premature P wave with no QRS response indicates a non-conducted premature atrial beat (PAB).

Bundle Branch Blocks (BBB)

A BBB is caused by a block in conduction within the right or left bundle branch. Remember that the bundle branches are a network of specialized conducting fibers, continuations of the AV bundle, which transmit electrical impulses in the ventricles. The blocked bundle branch delays depolarization to the ventricle that it supplies.

BBBs are characterized by a wide QRS complex (greater than 120 ms), usually resulting from disease of the bundle branches, or ventricular abnormalities. Drugs, electrolyte, or metabolic disorders can also cause BBBs. There are two classifications: right bundle branch block (RBBB) and left bundle branch block (LBBB). *Look at V_1 and V_6 to check for BBBs.*

> **RBBB**: Activation of the left ventricle occurs before the right ventricle. This causes a triphasic complex in lead V_1 (and often in V_2), which resembles *"rabbit ears."* When a RBBB is present, it should trigger screening for conditions that are affecting the right side of heart or lungs, including pulmonary emboli, COPD, and cardiomyopathy.
>
> **LBBB**: The initial QRS deflection is altered due to the initial impulse traveling across the septum from right to left. *This produces an initial negative deflection in V_1 and an initial upright deflection in V_6. Look for a wide, notched appearance.* Detection of a LBBB always needs to be followed up with an imaging study, because it usually indicates underlying cardiac pathology, including dilated or hypertrophic cardiomyopathy, hypertension, aortic valve disease, or cardiovascular disease.

Myocardial Ischemia

As previously mentioned, myocardial ischemia occurs with a decreased blood flow to the coronary arteries due to a partial or complete blockage. This reduces the heart's oxygen supply and can damage the heart muscle, reducing ability to pump effectively. Ischemia can also cause serious arrhythmias. Remember that ischemia is a warning sign; it is also, thankfully, reversible.

As a professional conducting exercise testing, especially with those who are at moderate to high risk for disease, you need to be comfortable with the **identification of ischemia**. Ischemia is evidenced in the ST-segment as a depression greater than or equal to 1 mm below the baseline. Both the magnitude and the character of the ST depression are important. Horizontal or down-sloping ST-segment depression is more specific for coronary artery disease than up-sloping ST depression.

Usually, the extent of ischemia is considered to be proportional to the degree of ST-segment depression, the number of ECG leads involved, and the duration of that depression in recovery.

Myocardial Infarction (MI)

Also known as a heart attack, myocardial infarction results from the near-total or complete blockage of an artery, which blocks blood flow to an area of the heart. Consider the MI Triad: ischemia, injury, and necrosis. Ischemia refers to the initial lack of oxygen, which spans over minutes. Injury refers to injury to the myocardium, which results from continued ischemia, (20 – 40 minutes). Eventually, **necrosis** occurs, which is death of the tissue. The timespan here is 2 – 12 hours.

Four ECG indicators of acute infarction are abnormal Q waves, ST segment depression, ST segment elevation, and T wave inversion. Be sure to scan ALL leads for these signs to determine location of infarct.

The abnormal Q waves (width greater than or equal to 1 small square, or 25% amplitude of R wave) represent necrosis. T waves often invert, and ST segments usually return to baseline in the days and weeks following an MI. Depending on the location and degree of heart damage, Q waves may be present.

MIs that don't feature Q waves or ST-segment elevation are called "non-STEMIs." MIs that do feature those characteristics are called "STEMIs." People with non-STEMI infarcts have a better short-term, but a worse long-term, prognosis than patients with STEMI.

Chamber Enlargement

Right Atrial Enlargement

Evidenced by a biphasic P wave, where the initial component is larger, right atrial enlargement is seen in leads V_1 and V_2. Look at the inferior leads (II, III, and aVF) for tall, peaked P waves. Remember: Normal P wave amplitude is < 2.5 mm.

This condition can accompany pathologies that affect the right side of the heart: COPD, congenital heart disease, coronary artery disease, pulmonary hypertension, pulmonary stenosis, tricuspid valve stenosis, tachycardia, or exercise.

Left Atrial Enlargement

This condition is evidenced by a biphasic P wave, where the second component is large and wide in V_1. Broad notched P waves in leads I and II can also indicate this condition. This condition can accompany pathologies that affect the left side of the heart: mitral valve disease, hypertension, aortic stenosis or regurgitation, or hypertrophic cardiomyopathy.

Right Ventricular Hypertrophy

Remember that **hypertrophy** is an increased thickness in tissue. Start by checking the R and S waves for hypertrophy. You will find height increases in R waves in lead V_1 (and sometimes in V_2). The R wave will become progressively smaller from $V_2 – V_6$.

If the R wave in lead V_1 has greater amplitude than the S wave, and the S wave in lead V_6 is has greater amplitude than the R wave, then right ventricular hypertrophy is indicated.

Left Ventricular Hypertrophy

The diagnostic criteria for this condition are: increased amplitude of the R wave in leads overlying the left ventricle (V_3-V_6), and increased amplitude of the S wave in leads overlying the right ventricle (V_1-V_2). You will also find – especially in the chest leads – that the QRS complexes will be exaggerated in amplitude, height, and depth.

Treatments for Cardiac Pathologies

Pacemakers

Pacemakers help the heart beat regularly at an appropriate rate, by assisting or replacing the heart's normal electrical conduction system. The most common cause for the need of a pacemaker is a slow heart rate. Typically, the indications include SA Node dysfunction and AV Block. Pacemakers can be identified on the ECG by unnaturally sharp spikes superimposed on the underlying rhythm. When the pacemaker fires, it produces a wave consistent with the chamber being paced.

There are several different types of pacemakers, each serving different physiologic purposes.

1. **Single-Chamber Pacemakers**:
    - Use one lead, either to the right atrium or right ventricle.
    - When the lead is placed in the ventricle, the pacemaker is able to receive signals from and pace *only the ventricle.*
    - If the lead is placed in the atrium, the pacemaker will be able to receive signals and pace *only the atrium.*
    - **On ECG**: For an atrial pacemaker, look for a spike followed by a P wave. For a ventricular pacemaker, look for a spike followed by wide, bizarre QRS complex.

2. **Dual-Chamber Pacemakers**:
    - Two leads, one to the right atrium and right ventricle each, provide AV synchrony.
    - These have lower mortality rates and higher survival rates.
    - **On ECG:** Look for two spikes in each cardiac cycle.

3. **Implantable Cardioverter Defibrillator (ICD)**:
    - The most common use for an ICD is a fast heart rate.
    - ICDs are indicated for sudden cardiac death due to: ventricular tachycardia or ventricular fibrillation with no reversible cause; spontaneous and sustained ventricular tachycardia; syncope without known cause; and non-sustained ventricular tachycardia with coronary artery disease.

Angiography
By injecting radio-opaque contrasting agent into the blood vessel (using a long, then catheter), this imaging technique allows the inside of blood vessels and heart chambers to be visualized – helping to identify any compromised artery openings, as well as the presence of atherosclerosis.

Cardiac Catheterization
In addition to serving interventional treatment purposes, this minimally-invasive procedure provides diagnostic information, identifying cardiac pathologies such as blockages, stenosis, thrombosis, etc.

One of the most common procedures done through cardiac catheterization is **angioplast**y, or the placement of stents. **Stents** are expandable stainless steel mesh tubes, which are placed in a vessel via balloon catheter to expand a blocked or stenotic artery; this allows blood flow.

Coronary Bypass Surgery
Sometimes the best option for treating heart disease is revascularization surgery, due to extensive atherosclerosis or blockage. This surgery restores blood flow to the heart by rerouting the flow of blood around a segment of a blocked artery in the heart. With this surgery, a healthy blood vessel is removed from another part of the body (usually an arm or leg). It is then connected to the arteries in the heart, "bypassing" the diseased/blocked area. This surgery can be done to a single artery, or multiple arteries. It improves symptoms such as angina and shortness of breath, both signs of poor blood flow in the heart.

Pharmacologic Agents
There are many different types of pharmacological agents, which are used to treat and manage heart disease. Be sure to know the classes of drugs, and their mechanisms of action. Here is a brief outline pertaining to the conditions discussed previously:

1. **Beta Blockers**: Decrease heart rate and cardiac output by blocking the effects of adrenaline on the heart.
    - Used for hypertension, angina, arrhythmias, MI, and heart failure.
    - Popular types: Metroprolol and Tenormin.

2. **Ace Inhibitors**: Expand blood vessels and lower resistance by lowering angiotensin II levels.
    - Used for hypertension and chronic heart failure.
    - Popular types: Lisinopril and Enalapril.

3. **Nitrates**: Relax the blood vessels and increase the blood and oxygen supply to the heart.
    - Used for angina and chronic heart failure. One of the first treatments applied when a patient presents ischemic symptoms, along with providing supplemental oxygen.
    - Popular types: Nitrostat and Imdur.

4. **Anti-Arrhythmics**: Work by either suppressing the activity of tissue that is initiating electrical impulses too quickly in SA Node, or by slowing and regulating the transmission of fast electrical impulses inside the heart.
    - Used to suppress atrial fibrillation; maintain a normal sinus rhythm; treat ventricular arrhythmias; and to slow the ventricular response in atrial fibrillation.
    - Popular types: Amiodarone and Norpace.

5. **Anti-Coagulants**: Decrease the clotting ability of the blood.
    - Used to treat atrial fibrillation.
    - Popular type: Coumadin.

Test Your Knowledge: Electrocardiography and Diagnostic Techniques

1. Which of the waveforms on the ECG will yield information about atrial enlargement? What should you look for?

2. In a third-degree AV block, how many impulses from the SA Node penetrate the AV node to depolarize the ventricles? Is the rhythm regular or irregular?

3. Which leads do you look for RBBB in? LBBB?

4. What are the characteristic ECG changes that yield information about ischemia?

5. What criteria need to be met for ST-segment elevation to be considered "abnormal" on an ECG? ST-segment depression?

6. Which part of the ECG will yield information about the AV Node?

7. True/False: sinus tachycardia is a regular rhythm.

8. What rhythm produces a straight line on the ECG, suggesting that there is no electrical activity left in the heart?

9. Cardiac muscle cells are unique in that they are able to generate their own electrical impulse. What is that ability called?

10. Leads V_3 and V_4 view which area of the heart?

11. On an ECG, what does the P wave represent?

Test Your Knowledge: Electrocardiography and Diagnostic Techniques – Answers

1. P waves yield information about atrial enlargement. You should look for tall, peaked P waves.

2. Remember, third-degree is a total block; therefore, there are **no** impulses from the SA Node penetrating the AV node. This is a regular rhythm.

3. For RBBB, look for leads V_1 and V_2. For LBBB, look for leads V_5 and V_6.

4. ECG changes such as **inverted T waves and/or ST-segment depression** yield information about ischemia.

5. In order to be considered "abnormal," an ST-segment must be greater than or equal to 1 mm *above* the baseline in two or more continuous leads. ST-segment depression occurs when the ST-segment is greater than or equal to 1 mm *below* the baseline in two or more continuous leads.

6. The PR-interval yields information about the AV Node – it will tell you the relationship between the atrial and ventricles.

7. **True**. Sinus tachycardia is a regular rhythm.

8. **Asystole**: A rhythm which produces a straight line on the ECG, suggestion no electrical activity in the heart.

9. **Automaticity**: The ability in cardiac muscle cells to generate their own electrical impulse.

10. Leads V_3 and V_4 view the **anterior left ventricle** of the heart.

11. The P wave represents **atrial depolarization** on an ECG.

References and Additional Reading

This chapter utilized the work of many outside texts, which you may also find useful as supplemental reading materials.

i. Dubin, D. (2000). *Rapid interpretation of EKG's* (V ed.). Tampa, FL: COVER Publishing Company.

ii. Ehrman, J. K. (2010). *ACSM's Resource manual for guidelines for exercise testing and prescription* (6th ed.). Baltimore, MD: Lippincott Williams & Wilkins.

iii. Thompson, W. R. (2010). *ACSM's Guidelines for exercise testing and prescription* (8th ed.). Baltimore, MD: Lippincott Williams & Wilkins.

Chapter 10: Medical and Surgical Management

Medical and surgical management refers to the coordination of health care services appropriate to achieve the goal of treatment and rehabilitation after a disease diagnosis. This management may include, but is not limited to, care assessment and assistance in developing, implementing, and coordinating a medical care plan with multiple healthcare providers, as well as the patient and his/her family.

Medical and surgical management requires evaluating a medical condition, developing and implementing a plan of care, coordinating medical resources, and communicating healthcare needs to the individual while monitoring and assisting in adherence to treatment.

Human Growth and Development

Human development is the process of growing to maturity. From a biological standpoint, human development is a continuum, starting with fertilization before going on to prenatal development, birth, and then further growth to adulthood. The age groups are as follows:

- Infancy: 3 weeks to 1 year.
- Childhood: 1 to 10 years.
- Juvenile: 10 to 16 years.
- Adolescence: 16 years to early 20s.
- Adulthood: Early 20s to 64 years.
- Senescence: 65 to 100 years and older.

A person's age must be considered when designing and implementing any type of structured exercise program.

Exercise for Children and Adolescents

Children and adolescents are perceived to be energetic, fit, and strong, because they are young. However, youths needs to develop good, consistent physical activity and sport habits so that they will be lifelong exercisers.

To achieve this, we need to educate children on the importance of staying active and on the impact of activity on their health and well-being. Keep in mind that children and young people have specific physical, physiological, and psychological capabilities that need to be considered when they participate in physical activity.

Considerations When Designing an Exercise Prescription

Physiological Considerations for Adolescents:

1. Higher maximal and submaximal oxygen uptake (VO2max)., resulting in increased oxygen delivery. This corresponds with growth spurt, resulting from hypertrophy of the heart and stimulation of red blood cells and hemoglobin.
2. Higher resting and exercising heart rates.
3. Lower resting and exercising blood pressures.
4. Hormonal changes.
5. Thermoregulatory differences, resulting in reduced sweating rate and higher heat production and increased sensitivity to excessive heat and cold.
6. Musculoskeletal and Bone Formation.
7. Body Composition.

The following considerations also need to be included:

Physical Considerations for Adolescents:

1. Existing medical conditions:
    - Asthma: A chronic respiratory disorder characterized by recurrent breathing difficulties and bronchial spasms; can be exacerbated by exercise.
    - Epilepsy: A common and diverse set of chronic neurological disorder characterized by seizures.
    - Diabetes: A chronic disease in which there are increased levels of sugar in the blood.
2. Overuse injuries due to: inadequate warm-up, improper footwear, poor technique, faulty equipment, or overtraining.
3. Appropriateness of resistance training:
    - Strict Supervision is required.
    - Sports/Activity Specific.
    - Focus on proper technique by starting with body weight resistance exercise (push-ups) and progressing to using light weights with frequent repetitions.

Psychological Considerations for Adolescents:

1. Healthy Body Image: Maintaining a healthy body image is one of the most important drivers of self-esteem among youth. Social pressures (from peers or others) often have a major role in shaping how our children view themselves. A healthy body image is a result of participation in healthy behaviors (healthy nutrition and regular physical activity) and acceptance of the idea that health, not appearance, is the main priority.

2. Mental Discipline (parents and coaches need to be on the lookout for the following states):

    - State anxiety: Stress reaction that occurs during sport/recreation preparation.

    - Trait anxiety: Intrinsic personality characteristic that may be compounded in situation stress (worry, self-criticism, and anxiety).

    - Burn-out: A reaction to the stresses of training and competition that manifests as emotional exhaustion, withdrawal, and decreased physical performance.

3. Social Skills: Giving children opportunities to play with others their age is one of the best ways to exercise social skills. While parents can create activities and games at home that help to teach them to act, they cannot anticipate the words and actions of other children. These interactions help to reinforce teamwork, effective communication, rule organization, and compromise.

4. Lifestyle Attitudes: Participation in sports and recreational physical activity has numerous benefits that can be seen in young age groups. It helps youth develop coping and decision making skills for the competitive world and teaches them how to attempt to achieve realistic personal goals. Structured activities set the foundation for challenges that help to motivate towards cooperation, and self-gratification.

Current research data does not allow recognition of a certain minimal level of daily physical activity; however, a reasonable goal is for children to engage in at least a moderate level of activity 30 - 60 minutes on most days of the week. As there are no evidence-based standard approaches to improving exercise habits in this demographic, the following models can be used:

1. Adult Prescription Model: Activity is performed for a number of minutes, 3 to 5 times a week. Examples: walking or biking.

2. Exercise "Menu:" A list of possible activities is presented, based off of the child's interest and the feasibility within the community. Examples: team sports, recreational activities, activity clubs.

3. Increasing Lifestyle Activities: No structured activity, simply an increase in everyday activities to increase caloric expenditure. Examples: using stairs instead of escalator or elevator, or walking or riding a bike instead of driving or being driven to a destination.

4. Decreasing Sedentary Time: Reducing the amount of time watching T.V or playing video games.

For children ages 5 to 12 an accumulation of at least 60 minutes, up to several hours, of age-appropriate activity on all or most days of the week is advised. Daily accumulation should be a combination of moderate and vigorous activity, intermittent in nature.

They should participate in several bouts of physical activity lasting 15 minutes or more each day. This participation needs a variety of age-appropriate activities that are designed to achieve optimal health, wellness, and performance benefits. Extended periods (2 hours or more) of inactivity are discouraged for children and adolescents, especially during daytime hours.

Exercise Prescription for Children & Adolescents:

Aerobic Activity:

- Frequency: 5 - 7 days a week.
- Intensity: Moderate to vigorous activity that is intermittent in nature.
- Time: 60 minutes or more/day; should be in several sessions of 15 - 20 minutes.
- Type: Age-appropriate exercise that utilizes all muscle groups (running, swimming, etc.).

Resistance Training:

- Frequency: 5 - 7 days a week.
- Intensity: 4 - 6 muscle groups; 1 - 3 sets of 8 - 15 repetitions for each group.
- Time: 20 - 30 minutes for each session. Add weight gradually up to a max of 6 reps; add 1 - 2 reps per session up to a max of 12 - 15 reps.
- Type: Submaximal resistance; make use of full range of motion.

Flexibility Activity:

- Frequency: 5 - 7 days a week.
- Intensity: Light to moderate; 12 -13 on the Borg scale.
- Time: Each stretch should be held for 15 - 30 seconds.
- Type: 2 - 4 static stretches for each muscle group.

Exercise for Older Adults

The majority of adults become less physically active with age, increasing their risk of developing a number of chronic disease states. Reports indicate that only about 21% of people aged 65 and older engage in regular activity. Evidence supports that the benefits of exercise in this age group include:

- Slowing physiological age changes that decrease exercise capacity.
- Optimizing age-related changes in body composition.
- Improving psychological and cognitive well-being.
- Managing of chronic disease.
- Reducing risk of physical impairment and increasing longevity.

A comprehensive pre-exercise evaluation in a clinical setting is recommended, which generally includes a medical history, physical exam, and variety of laboratory tests to identify:

- Medical contraindications to exercise.
- Risks of disease where exercise testing is needed prior to starting an exercise program.
- Clinical significant disease states that would require an individual to participate in a medically supervised exercise programs.
- Special needs and considerations.

Physiological Considerations:

1. Lower maximum and sub-maximum oxygen uptake, due to reduced maximum heart rate and cardiac output.
2. Higher resting and exercising blood pressures.
3. Decreased immune function.
4. Decreased sensitivity in thermoregulation, resulting in reduced total body water and reduced capacity for sweating.
5. Increase in risk factors, such as:
    - Hypertension: High blood pressure.
    - Hyperlipidemia: Increased blood cholesterol levels.
    - Diabetes: A chronic disease in which there are increased levels of sugar in the blood.
    - Coronary artery disease: A narrowing of the small blood vessels that supply blood and oxygen to the heart.

Physical Considerations:

1. Decrease in bone and muscle mass.

2. Decreased balance and coordination.

3. Increase in obesity; higher percentage of fat mass.

4. Osteoarthritis:_degenerative arthritis or degenerative joint disease.

5. Orthopedic injuries.

Psychological Considerations:

1. Self-efficacy: Research shows that exercise improves many older adults' perception of their ability to perform the tasks needed to achieve personal goals. Evidence further shows that this improvement in self-efficacy is critical for decreasing functional decline and impairment.

2. Self-concept: The way one sees themselves, or their self-esteem, is based on feelings of being valued, useful, and competent. Changes in roles, activities, and lifestyles that often occur with aging may cause a change in self-esteem.

3. Cognitive functioning: Physical fitness has beneficial effects on cognitive functioning.

4. Life satisfaction: Older adults who exercise regularly tend to demonstrate a more positive attitude toward work and are generally healthier. There is also a strong correlation between activity levels and self-reported happiness.

Exercise Prescription Guidelines for Older Adults

Aerobic Activity:

- Frequency: 5 - 7 days a week.

- Intensity: Light to moderate; 50 - 80% of maximum HR.

- Time: 30 - 60 minutes a day (can be in 10 - 15 minute intervals).

- Type: Walking, stationary bicycling; low orthopedic stress.

Resistance Training: [23]

- Frequency: 2 days a week.

- Intensity: 1 set of 8 - 10 repetitions for each muscle group; Borg scale: 12 - 13.

- Time: 20 - 30 minutes a session; add weight gradually as tolerated.

- Type: Weight training machines; tubing & bands (with assistance).

---

[23] Older adults should be discouraged from strength/resistance training during active periods of pain or inflammation.

Flexibility Activity:

- Frequency: 5 - 7 days a week.
- Intensity: Light to moderate; 12 - 13 on the Borg scale.
- Time: Each stretch should be held for 15 - 30 seconds.
- Type: 2 - 4 static stretches for each muscle group.

Diseases: Factors and Treatments

In order to maximize the effectiveness of medical and surgical management, having a solid understanding of a variety of chronic diseases is essential. Knowing the risk factors and treatments for the following conditions helps health fitness professionals, at all levels, to prevent, diagnose, manage, and treat with competence.

Chronic Obstructive Pulmonary Disease (COPD) is a group of lung diseases that block airflow as you exhale. Individuals with COPD experience shortness of breath, or **dyspnea**, due to this difficulty in exhaling all the air out from their lungs. The main conditions are:

1. Emphysema: A condition that damages the alveoli by destroying the inner walls and making them weaker and less elastic. This reduces the surface area for oxygen exchange.
2. Chronic asthmatic bronchitis: Chronic inflammation and narrowing of the airways leading to the lungs, causing coughing and wheezing.
3. Asthma: A chronic breathing disorder characterized by frequent bronchospasms.
4. Cystic Fibrosis: In most cases, the symptoms of COPD do not appear until there is significant lung damage and continue to worsen over time. Symptoms include shortness of breath, wheezing, chest tightness, and chronic coughing. COPD is a leading cause of death and disability, with the most common cause being smoking. Age and occupational exposure to dust and chemicals are also key risk factors.

If COPD is suspected, the following tests may be used for diagnosis:

- Chest X-ray.
- Computerized Tomography (CT).
- Arterial blood gas analysis: Measures how well your lungs are bringing oxygen into your blood and removing carbon dioxide.
- Sputum examination: Analysis of the cells found in mucus helps to rule out lung cancer or a bacterial infection.
- Pulmonary Function Test (PFT): A post bronchodilator ration of FEV1 (forced expiratory volume in 1 second) / FVC (forced vital capacity) of ≤ 0.7 is indicative of nonreversible airflow limitation.

Since the damage is irreversible, treatments focus on controlling symptoms and minimizing damage to improve quality of life. Quitting smoking is an essential step in the treatment plan as it is the only way to stop COPD from progressing.

Medications, such as bronchodilators, inhaled steroids, and antibiotics are used to assist in symptom relief.

Other forms of therapy include supplemental oxygen and pulmonary rehabilitation. There are also surgical treatments for individuals with severe emphysema:

- Lung volume reduction surgery: a small wedge of damaged lung tissue is removed. This creates extra space in the chest cavity for the remaining lung tissue and diaphragm to work more efficiently.

- Lung transplant.

Restrictive Lung Disease is a group of lung diseases characterized by restriction in the lungs causing the inability to fully inhale. This results from conditions causing stiffness in the lungs, the chest wall, weak muscles, or nerve damage. These conditions include:

- Interstitial lung disease/Pulmonary Fibrosis: A group of lung diseases affecting the interstitium (the tissue and space around the air sacs of the lungs).

- Sarcoidosis: A disease that results from a specific type of inflammation of tissues of the body. It can appear in almost any body organ, but it starts most often in the lungs or lymph nodes.

- Obesity: Excessive body fat.

- Scoliosis: An abnormal curvature of the lumbar spine.

- Muscular Dystrophy or Amyotrophic Lateral Sclerosis (ALS): A group of inherited disorders that involve muscle weakness and loss of muscle tissue.

Restrictive Lung Diseases restrict and reduce lung volume and tidal volume due to one, or all of the following: loss of functioning of the alveoli-capillary unit, altered mechanical function of the thorax and pulmonary system, or secondary cardiovascular dysfunction. The same diagnostic tests that are used to diagnose COPD are also used to diagnose restrictive lung diseases and according to the National Institute of Health, the following treatments can also be utilized:

- Immunosuppressant drugs (*Imuran, Cytoxan, Rheumatrex, Trexall*): These keep your immune system from attacking and destroying healthy tissue. They also can be used to slow or stop the growth of abnormal tissue or cells.

- Corticosteroids (inhaled or oral): These can reduce swelling and inflammation and suppress the immune system so it doesn't attack healthy cells.

- Anti-inflammatory drugs: Reducing inflammation and swelling can ease symptoms.

- Anti-fibrotic drugs: These investigational drugs may slow or stop extra tissue from forming on the lungs.

Individuals diagnosed with either intrinsic (internal causes) or extrinsic (external causes) restrictive lung disease can also benefit from oxygen therapy and pulmonary rehabilitation.

Cardiovascular Disease (CVD) refers to any disease that affects the cardiovascular system, especially cardiac disease, vascular diseases of the brain and kidney, and peripheral arterial disease.

According to the American College of Sports Medicine and the American College of Cardiology, there are multiple non-modifiable and modifiable risk factors for the development of cardiovascular disease.

Non-modifiable Risk Factors: Advancing age, gender, and family history.

Modifiable Risk Factors: Tobacco smoking, dyslipidemia, hypertension, physical inactivity, overweight/obesity, diabetes (type 2), and metabolic syndrome.

Diabetes: Diabetes is a group of metabolic diseases in which a person has high blood sugar, either because the pancreas does not produce enough insulin (Type I or IDDM), or because cells do not respond to the insulin that is produced (Type II or NIDDM) . The risk factors for diabetes depend on disease etiology. The primary risk factor for the development of Type I diabetes is family history, especially if one has a parent or sibling with the disease.

Injury or diseases of the pancreas can inhibit its ability to produce insulin and lead to Type 1 diabetes, as can a range of relatively rare infections and illnesses, and risk factors for Type II diabetes include:

- Obesity/Overweight.
- Ethnicity.
- Insulin resistance.
- Hypertension.
- Family History.
- Sedentary Lifestyle.
- Age.

Even with recent breakthroughs and advancements in science and technology, there is currently no cure for diabetes. Keeping the level of glucose in the blood within the normal range, however, can control it. Patients with Type I diabetes can be treated with insulin several times a day, while patients with Type II diabetes may not need insulin.

Diabetes in these patients is typically controlled with diet and physical activity, as well as oral hypoglycemic agents such as *Metformin, Glucophage*, and *Glucotrol.* In cases where glucose levels are not well controlled with oral glycemics, some Type II patients find that they do need to be placed on insulin therapy.

Edema is swelling that is caused by fluid trapped in the body's tissues. Edema happens most often in the feet, ankles, and legs, but can affect other parts of the body, such as the face, hands, and abdomen. Signs and symptoms include:

- Swelling or puffiness of the tissue directly under the skin.
- Stretched or shiny skin.
- Skin that retains "pitting" after being pressed.
- Increased abdominal size.

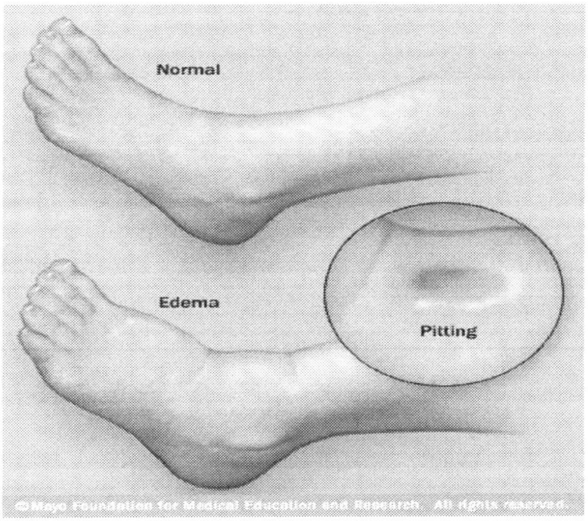

Certain diseases such as congestive heart failure and lung, liver, kidney, and thyroid diseases are significant risk factors as they can cause edema or make it worse. Edema can also be exacerbated by certain medications for blood pressure, diabetes, or pain. Allergic reactions, severe inflammation, burns, trauma, clot(s), or poor nutrition can also cause edema. Edema can be temporary or permanent, depending on its cause and is treated according to the condition that is causing it. For example, if edema is caused by lung disease, such as emphysema or chronic bronchitis, quitting smoking is advised. For patients with chronic heart failure, treating coronary artery disease; monitoring weight, fluid, and salt intake and cutting down on excess alcohol would be recommended.

Signs and Symptoms of Cardiopulmonary and Metabolic Diseases:

1. Pain or discomfort in the chest, neck, jaw, or back.
2. Resting or mild exertional dyspnea.
3. Dizziness or syncope.
4. Paroxysmal nocturnal dyspnea.
5. Orthopnea (inability to breathe while lying down).
6. Ankle edema.
7. Palpitations (sensation of a "skipped" beat) or rapid heart rate.
8. Claudication.
9. Heart murmurs.
10. Unusual fatigue or dyspnea with activities of daily living (ADL's).

Metabolic Syndrome
According to the American Heart Association (AHA) and the Adult Treatment Panel III (ATP III), a group of metabolic risk factors in an individual characterizes the metabolic syndrome. These risk factors are described as follows:

1. Central Obesity: Excessive adipose tissue in and around the abdomen as measured by waist circumference. For men: greater than 40 inches. For women: greater than 35 inches.

2. Atherogenic Dyslipidemia: Blood fat disorders, mainly high triglycerides and low high-density lipid (HDL) cholesterol, which fosters plaque build-up in the artery walls. A fasting blood triglyceride greater than or equal to 150mg/dL is present with blood HDL cholesterol levels. For men: less than 40mg/dL. For women: less than 50mg/dL

3. Insulin Resistance/Glucose Intolerance: defined as when the body cannot properly use insulin or glucose with a fasting blood glucose greater than or equal to 110mg/dL. Insulin resistance is present in a majority of individuals with metabolic syndrome, since it strongly associates with other metabolic risk factors. Patients with longstanding insulin resistance frequently manifest glucose intolerance, another emerging risk factor.

4. Proinflammatory State: elevated high-sensitivity C-reactive protein in the blood. There are multiple mechanisms that appear to underlie elevation of CRP, including obesity, as excessive adipose tissue releases inflammatory cytokines that may elicit higher CRP levels.

5. Prothrombic State: increased fibrinogen or plasminogen activator inhibitor [-1] in the blood. Fibrinogen, an acute-phase reactant similar to CRP, rises in response to a high-cytokine state.

6. Hypertension: an elevated blood pressure of 130/85mmHg (or higher) strongly associates with obesity and insulin resistance, even though it is considered to be multifactorial in origin.

Effects of Exercise on Pulmonary Disorders
The benefits of exercise through pulmonary rehabilitation are seen even in irreversible pulmonary disorders, because much of the disability and handicap results not from the disorder itself, but from secondary morbidities that are often treatable if recognized. Although the degree of airway obstruction or hyperinflation of chronic obstructive pulmonary disease (COPD) does not change appreciably with pulmonary rehabilitation, reversal of muscle deconditioning and better pacing enable patients to walk farther and with less dyspnea.

Several impairments, such as weakness, dysfunction of peripheral and respiratory muscles, anxiety and depression, and abnormalities of nutrition, have responded to treatment. Improvements in overall and exertional dyspnea, as well as health-related quality of life (QOL) measures, have been documented. Significant increases in maximal exercise capacity, as measured during exercise testing, have been observed. As pulmonary disease is commonly associated with coronary artery disease (CAD) and CAD risk factors, exercise training also helps reduce the risk of CAD in individuals with pulmonary disorders (ACSM).

Effects of Exercise on Asthma
Research has shown that exercise triggers bronchial narrowing in asthma by bringing large volumes of air deep into the chest. At rest or with light activities, the air that enters the lungs is warmed and moisturized by the nose, mouth and throat. By the time the air reaches the bronchial tubes inside the

chest, it has nearly the same temperature and moisture as the walls of the bronchial tubes themselves. During moderate to vigorous exercise, one's level of breathing may double or triple, decreasing one's ability to warm and humidify completely the inspired air. In asthma, this loss of heat and moisture from the walls of the bronchial tubes makes them contract, causing wheezing and coughing.

Several strategies can be used to prevent symptoms of asthma after exercise. On a cold day, trap a little bit of warm, moist air in front of the mouth by using a scarf pulled up over the nose and mouth. For serious athletes, a warm-up period of light exertion can help to reduce symptoms during competition. Medications taken before exercise are effective in blocking asthmatic symptoms. One or two puffs of a prescribed beta-agonist bronchodilator (for example, *albuterol*) inhaled ten minutes before exercise usually prevents exercise-induced asthma.

Effects of Exercise on the Metabolic Syndrome

The constellation of hypertension, dyslipidemia, impaired glucose tolerance, insulin insensitivity, and central obesity is recognized in the medical community as the metabolic syndrome. This syndrome will likely soon overtake cigarette smoking as the number one risk factor for heart and other chronic disease states among the U.S. population. While a healthy diet plan with judicious use of medications has been recommended to address specific risk factors, research has shown that all forms of physical activity, acute and chronic, have a substantial impact on these components:

1. Hypertension. There is a significant amount of evidence that aerobic training helps to reduce blood pressure and SBP.

2. Dyslipidemia. Low saturated fat diets combined with exercise lower total cholesterol, LDL-C, and triglyceride concentrations, while increasing HDL-C levels. Alternatively, nutritional supplements combined with exercise, decreased total cholesterol, LDL-C, and triglyceride concentrations, while increasing HDL-C levels. Combinations of lifestyle therapies, including exercise, are effective in improving cholesterol levels.

3. Glucose Intolerance/Insulin Insensitivity. Beneficial effects of exercise on insulin sensitivity have been demonstrated in acute bouts, as well as in longer periods, of physical activity. Short-term effects are detectable even after a single session of exercise and are mediated mostly by the metabolic changes in insulin signaling inside the muscle tissue.

   Modifications in fatty acid metabolism related to a decrease in intracellular accumulation of intermediary metabolites interfering with insulin signaling have been shown to have a strong impact on improved muscle insulin sensitivity. Chronic exercise has been shown to lead to an improved glucose tolerance.

4. Obesity. Exercise is essential in the treatment of obesity. However, one of the most marked disabilities arising from obesity is a reduced exercise tolerance, so severely obese patients are unable to perform the exercises which would bring these benefits. Obesity is best treated by a combination of dietary restriction and exercise; the more severe the obesity the more important the dietary component of treatment, while exercise is more important with the management of mild obesity or the prevention of obesity.

Effects of Exercise on Diabetes

Type I Diabetes (Insulin Dependent) affects the body's ability to use sugars, starches, fats, and proteins. Because the body needs various fuels for energy, this disease disrupts normal energy metabolism both at rest and during physical exercise.

Following digestion, a hormone called insulin is released into the blood from the pancreas. Among insulin's primary roles is its ability to allow carbohydrates (absorbed in the form of glucose) and proteins to enter muscle cells, where they are stored or used for energy. Individuals with type 1 diabetes are unable to produce enough—or even any—insulin to allow this process to occur. Consequently, glucose is unable to enter cells and builds up in the blood.

Because people with type 1 diabetes have insufficient insulin production, daily insulin injections are required to maintain glucose levels as close to normal as possible. Thus, individuals with type 1 diabetes are considered insulin-dependent. It is imperative for those with type 1 diabetes to regulate their blood glucose (blood sugar) levels to help reduce complications associated with this disease.

If glucose levels remain unchecked for extended periods, people with type 1diabetes run the risk of developing heart disease, kidney failure, blindness, and nerve dysfunction.

Exercise uses glucose as a fuel, so it is an effective way to control blood sugar levels. Exercise has an insulin-like effect on glucose, enhancing its uptake into cells and counteracting elevated blood glucose levels that frequently occur after eating. With exercise, the amount of insulin injected for controlling blood glucose can be lowered in those with type 1 diabetes.

Type II Diabetes (Non-insulin Dependent) is characterized by a failure of insulin to remove glucose from the bloodstream. Under healthy conditions, insulin interacts with body cell mechanisms that permit the passage of glucose out of blood circulation and into tissues. Impairment of this process, called insulin resistance, results in hyperglycemia, type 2 diabetes, and other health problems.

A single episode of exercise helps insulin clear glucose from circulation for 12 to 48 hours after exercise. Regular episodes of physical activity sustain this effect, minimizing hyperglycemic consequences over time. Improvements in glucose control result from adaptations of skeletal muscles to physical training, because these muscles use glucose to power physical activity.

Taxing muscles increases their need for glucose, and regular training increases glucose storage capacity, generates new blood vessels within muscles, and improves insulin's ability to push glucose into cells.

Effects of Exercise on Coronary Artery Disease

The mechanisms responsible for a decrease in coronary artery disease vary and include:

1. The effects of exercise on CAD risk factors:

    - Decrease in resting and exercise blood pressures.
    - Decrease in total cholesterol, LDL cholesterol, and triglyceride levels.
    - Increase in HDL cholesterol.
    - Improved glucose tolerance and insulin sensitivity.
    - Decrease in body fat percentage and waist circumference.

2. A reduction in cardiac oxygen demand at rest and at submaximal workloads, leading to an increase in ischemic/angina thresholds.

3. A reduction in platelet aggregation.

4. An improvement in endothelial function and tone.

The following classes of medications are frequently used in the treatment of CAD; therefore, knowing how they respond to exercise is crucial when performing diagnostic tests and prescribing exercise therapy.

1. **Angiotensin-Converting Enzyme (ACE) inhibitors**: Used to treat hypertension, these act by reducing myocardial oxygen demand through reducing vascular resistance. They may increase exercise tolerance in those with left ventricular dysfunction and reduce resting and exercising blood pressure. Examples: *Atacand, Avapro, Cozaar, Micardis, Diovan, Benicar.*

2. **Beta Adrenergic Blockers:** Used to treat hypertension, left ventricular dysfunction, and angina, these reduce ischemia, by decreasing oxygen demand, and controls ventricular dysrhythmias. They reduce resting and exercising heart rates and blood pressures and may increase exercise tolerance in those with ventricular dysfunction. Examples: *Toprol, Tenormin, Corgard, Inderal*

3. **Calcium Channel Antagonists**: Used to treat hypertension, angina, atrial fibrillation and supraventricular tachycardia, these reduce ischemia by altering the determinants of oxygen supply and demand. They reduce resting and exercising blood pressures, some may reduce resting and exercising heart rates. Examples: *Cardizem, Calan, Calan SR, Covera HS, Verelan PM.*

4. **Nitrates:** Used to treat angina and as a vasodilator in heart failure, these reduce ischemia by decreasing oxygen demand and by allowing a small increase in oxygen supply and decrease resting and exercising blood pressures. They are available in short and long-lasting forms. Examples: *Imdur, Nitrostat, Nitroquick, Nitrobid.*

5. **Digitalis:** Used for congestive heart failure, these enhance myocardial contractility, increasing stroke volume, and blunt SA and AV node conduction, reducing resting and exercising heart rates in those with tachycardia and atrial fibrillation. Example: *Digitalis.*

6. **Diuretics:** Used for mild hypertension, these reduce blood pressure by increasing renal secretion of sodium and potassium, resulting in a loss of water in the urine, mildly affecting resting and exercising blood pressures. They may increase exercise tolerance in patients with congestive heart failure. There are several types:
   - Thiazides: *Hydrochlorothiazide, Indapamide.*
   - Loop: *Bumex, Lasix.*
   - Potassium-sparing: *Midamor.*
   - Aldosterone receptor blockers: *Inspra, Aldactone.*
   - Combination diuretics: *Moduretic, Maxzide,*

Key Terms and Definitions

Claudication: Pain, tension, and weakness in the legs when walking, which intensifies to produce lameness and is relieved by rest. Claudication is a common symptom in peripheral artery disease (PAD).

Dyspnea: Labored breathing; is often associated with pulmonary disease and coronary artery disease.

Ischemia: An intermediate condition in CAD, during which the heart tissue is slowly or suddenly starved of oxygen and other nutrients. Eventually, the affected heart tissue will die. When blood flow is completely blocked to the heart, ischemia can lead to a heart attack. Ischemia can be silent or symptomatic, and up to four million Americans may have silent ischemia, putting them at high risk of having a heart attack with no warning.

Angina: "Discomfort" localized in the chest, caused by an insufficient supply of blood to the heart.

Embolism: An obstruction in a blood vessel due to a blood clot or other foreign matter that gets stuck while traveling through the bloodstream. Plural: emboli.

Stenosis: An abnormal narrowing or contraction of a valve or artery.

Tachycardia: An abnormally rapid heart rate. There are multiple types of tachycardia, depending on the place of impulse origin.

1. Sinus Tachycardia: Increased rate of electrical impulse originating from the SA node at > 100bpm.

2. Atrial Tachycardia: Has a more or less regular heart rate, of > 100 beats per minute, with narrow QRS complexes with P-waves that do not originate from the sinus node, but from another site in the atria.

3. Ventricular Tachycardia: A potentially life-threatening arrhythmia, with a heart rate of more than 100 beats per minute, with at least three irregular heartbeats in a row, which originates in one of the ventricles of the heart. May lead to ventricular fibrillation, asystole, and death.

It is important to know which electrocardiographic patterns and changes can occur in certain disorders and special populations. Their criteria are as follows:

1. Coronary Artery Disease (CAD): A horizontal or downward sloping ST depression of at least 1mm in 2 leads can signify CAD. T-wave abnormalities may also be seen.

2. Pulmonary Disease: Individuals with chronic COPD (i.e. emphysema) often exhibit low voltage QRS complexes and poor R-wave progression in the precordial leads, and may also exhibit a vertical, or rightward, axis.

3. Hypertensive Heart Disease: Left ventricular hypertrophy and left atrial enlargement are common. Also, left Bundle Branch Block (LBBB) and atrial fibrillation can occur.

4. Myocardial Ischemia and Infarction (MI): Ischemia can occur transiently and can affect the inner layer (subendocardium) or the entire ventricular wall (transmural). Infarction occurs when there is severe or prolonged ischemia.

- Localizations of Infarctions in corresponding ECG leads:
    - Anterior: Q waves in V1-V4.
    - Inferior: Q waves in II, III, and aVF..
    - Lateral: Q waves in I, aVL, V5, and V6.
    - Posterior: Tall R waves in V1-V2.

- Transmural Ischemia with MI:
    - Associated with changes in both QRS and ST complexes.
    - Early sign: ST elevation or tall, upright T waves.
    - Q waves begin to form within a few hours.
    - ST elevation may return to baseline and T waves become inverted.
    - Q waves may persist for years with T wave inversion persisting indefinitely.

- Subendocardial Ischemia with MI:
    - Usually produces ST segment depression in anterior and/or inferior leads during anginal attacks.
    - Marked by persistent ST depression, possible T wave inversion, and usually normal Q waves.

- Q- wave and Non-Q-wave Myocardial Infarction (QWMI vs. NQWMI).
    - NQWMI: Present with chest pain, enzyme evidence, but lacks Q-wave development on the ECG.
    - QWMI: Demonstrated and diagnosed by Q-waves on the surface ECG.

5. Atrial Enlargement. Left atrial: A wide P wave of > 0.12 seconds, best seen in V1. Commonly seen in mitral valve disease. Right atrial: A tall P wave amplitude > 2.5mm, best seen in II. Commonly seen in pulmonary disease. Biatrial: P wave may be “notched” or “biphasic” in morphology.

6. Ventricular Hypertrophy: Produces high voltage criteria in the leads over the hypertrophied areas.

- Left Ventricular Hypertrophy (LVH):
    - Associated with tall R waves in the left chest leads and deep S waves in the right chest leads.
    - S wave in V1 + R in V5 or V6 > 35mm or R wave in a VL > 11mm.
    - ST changes with T wave inversions are usually present in leads with tall R waves.
    - Commonly seen with aortic stenosis and hypertensive heart disease.

- Right Ventricular Hypertrophy (RVH):
    - High voltage criteria in V1 and V2 and possibly and R-wave greater than the S-wave in those leads.
    - Right axis deviation and ST changes with T-wave inversions.

7. Pericarditis: Associated with global ST segment elevation, pericarditis causes inflammation of the pericardium of the heart and can be followed by T-wave inversion.

8. Electrolyte Abnormalities:

- Hypokalemia: Decreased blood potassium levels.
    - ECG demonstrates ST depression with prominent U waves and flattened T waves.

- Hyperkalemia: Increased blood potassium levels.
    - Mild hyperkalemia: Narrow and peaked T waves.
    - Moderate hyperkalemia: Prolonged PR intervals and small or absent P waves.
    - Severe hyperkalemia: Wide QRS complexes and asystole.

- Hypocalcemia: Decreased blood calcium levels.
    - ECG demonstrates prolonged QT intervals.
    - Normal QT = 0.36 seconds.
    - QT = 0.48 seconds.

- Hypercalcemia: increased blood calcium levels.
    - ECG demonstrates shortened QT intervals.
    - Normal QT = 0.36 seconds.
    - QT = 0.26 seconds.

Health Behavior Adherence

Adherence is the single most important modifiable factor that compromises treatment outcomes, regardless of the disease. Therefore, each disease management plan should be formulated as an individualized therapeutic alliance among the patient and family, the physician, and other members of the health care team. Adherence is a multifaceted behavioral process determined by several factors. Key characteristics that can attribute to poor adherence are:

1. Lack of knowledge and skills about the health problem and self-regulation behaviors required, their mechanisms of action, and the importance of adherence.

2. Beliefs: The perceived severity and susceptibility (relevance), self-efficacy, outcome expectations, and response costs.

3. Motivation: Value and reinforcement, internal attribution of success (positive outcomes are reinforcing, negative results are an indication to modify behavior).

4. Action: Stimulated by relevant cues, driven by information recall, evaluation, and selection of behavioral options and available resources.

A plan should recognize self-management education as an integral component of care.

A variety of strategies and techniques should be used to provide adequate education and development of problem-solving skills in the various aspects of the individuals' lifestyle management, which can assist in behavior adherence:

1. Assess the individual's specific education needs.

2. Identify the individual's specific self-management goals.

3. Plan the teaching-learning and behavioral change process.

4. Implement the educational and behavioral intervention to help the individual achieve self-management goals.

5. Evaluate the individual's attainment of self-management goals.

ACSM recommends a three-function model of participant-centered education and counseling, as follows:

1. Information Gathering by the Health Professional:

    - Current level of knowledge.
    - Attitudinal beliefs, intentions, and readiness to change.
    - Previous experience with behavior change.
    - Behavioral skills.
    - Available social support.

2. Develop a helping relationship by establishing support:

    - Interactive communication with a willingness to negotiate.
    - Exhibit a non-judgmental attitude towards patient.
    - Establish support by exhibiting empathy, legitimizing concerns, respecting one's abilities and efforts, providing reinforcement and follow-ups, partnering with the individual, and paying attention to nonverbal communication.

3. Participant education and counseling: Participants in the earlier stages of change benefit most from cognitive strategies (lectures, books, etc.), while those in later stages depend more on behavioral techniques (reminders and the development of social support).During each session, the "Five A's" should be used:

    - Address the agenda.
    - Assess.
    - Advice.
    - Assist.
    - Arrange follow-up.

Poor adherence continues, because it is a complex problem and can be resistant to generic approaches. In situations in which patients are required to administer their own treatments (i.e. medications, nutrition, and exercise) non-adherence is likely, and the risk of non-adherence needs to be assessed as part of the treatment-planning process.

Volume Changes
A majority of clinical medicine consists of estimating the volume status of patients. Discussions about whether patients are "wet" or "dry" are a constant focus. The wet patients are often treated with diuretics, dialysis, or fluid restriction, whereas the dry ones receive intravenous fluids or blood transfusions. The clinical assessment of volume status relies mostly on indirect indicators, such as blood pressure, lung sounds, edema, jugular vein distension, changes in weight, input/output monitoring, and blood urea nitrogen/creatinine. Sometimes physicians must use a fluid challenge or invasive central pressure monitoring to assess volume status in a difficult patient. The importance of volume is also relevant to treatment mechanisms when it comes to assessing the lung volume, cardiac output, and body mass index

A plethysmograph is an instrument for measuring changes in volume within an organ or entire body, usually resulting from fluctuations in the amount of blood or air Within it. This is used in two main types of testing:

1. **Whole-body Plethysmography**: A technique that measures the volume of gas in the lungs, including that which is trapped in poorly communicating air spaces, of particular use in COPD and emphysema.

2. **Impedance Plethysmography** (Venous impedance plethysmography): A technique used to diagnose acute venous obstruction or vascular insufficiency of an extremity by measuring the change in limb volume with each arterial pulse and during cuff occlusion of the venous flow from the limb, the manipulation of which allows evaluation of either the arterial or venous flow.

Diagnostic Tests for Coronary Artery Disease
Diagnostic exercise testing is used in a clinical manner to assess a patient's ability to tolerate increasing intensities of exercise, or "stress", while monitoring ECG, hemodynamic, and symptomatic responses. These tests are used frequently in patients with an intermediate probability of significant cardiovascular disease (CVD), based on the theory that these patients will have marked ST segment depression on the ECG while exercising. There are several types of exercise stress tests that are utilized, depending on age, gender, and symptoms:

2. **Treadmill and Bike Exercise Tests**: Workload (work rate) is changed every 3 minutes by increasing the speed and incline on the treadmill or the resistance on the bike. Patients exercise until they are fatigued, develop symptoms, reach greater than 85% of their age-predicted maximum heart rate (MPHR), or symptoms occur. Symptoms to indicate early termination include, but are not limited to:

    - Moderately severe chest discomfort.
    - Marked shortness of breath.
    - Dizziness.
    - Drop in systolic blood pressure, > 10mmHg from baseline despite an increase in workload, accompanied by other signs of ischemia.
    - Signs of poor perfusion (cyanosis, pallor).

- Sustained ventricular tachycardia.
- ST elevation (+1mm) in leads without diagnostic Q-waves (other than V1 or a VR).
- Patients request to stop.

3. **Stress Tests with Myocardial Perfusion Imaging**:

- Myocardial Perfusion Imaging (MPI): A type of nuclear medicine procedure where a small amount of a radioactive substance, called a radionuclide (radioactive tracer), is used to assist in the examination of cardiac tissue. Specifically, the myocardial perfusion scan evaluates the heart's function and blood flow. A radionuclide is a radioactive substance used as a "tracer," which means it travels through the blood stream and is absorbed by the healthy heart muscle tissue. On the scan, the areas where the radionuclide has been absorbed will show up differently than the areas that do not absorb it, due to possible damage to the tissue from decreased or blocked blood flow.

- Exercise Stress MPI: Exercise is started at a slower "warm-up" speed. The speed of the treadmill and its slope or inclination is increased every 3 minutes. The treadmill workload is decreased for cool down when the patient exceeds 85% of their target heart rate (based upon the patient's age). Exercise may be stopped earlier if the patient develops signs or symptoms. This is used to determine what areas of the myocardium demonstrate decreased blood flow during peak exercise. This is done by injecting a radionuclide (thallium or technetium) into a vein in the arm or hand during exercise. After the radionuclide has been injected into a vein and has circulated through the blood stream, a special machine, called a gamma camera, takes pictures of the heart while the person lies still on a table. This scanning usually lasts about 15 - 30 minutes, depending on the camera. Rest images are completed prior to exercise. The resting phase is done in order to compare the results with the exercise phase to see if areas that do not get adequate blood flow while exercising are able to absorb the radionuclide during rest.

- Pharmacologic MPI: Used when it has been determined that exercise on a treadmill is not an appropriate choice, due to the person's medical condition. In this situation, a medication (*Lexiscan, Adenosine, or Persantine*) is given that causes the coronary arteries to dilate. This dilation of the coronary arteries causes an increase in blood flow that is similar to the response of the arteries during exercise. Rest images are completed prior to medication administration. The resting phase is done in order to compare the results with the stress phase to see if areas that do not get adequate blood flow are able to absorb the radionuclide during rest.

4. **Stress Echocardiography**:

- Echocardiography: Routinely used in the diagnosis, management, and follow-up of patients with any suspected or known heart diseases. It can provide the size and shape of the heart (internal chamber size quantification), pumping capacity, and the location and extent of any tissue damage. An echocardiogram can also give physicians other estimates of heart function, such as a calculation of the cardiac output, ejection fraction, and diastolic function (how well the heart relaxes).

- Exercise Stress Echocardiography: A resting study is completed, which provides a baseline examination and demonstrates the size and function of various chambers of the heart. Focus is on the patient's resting ejection fraction (EF), a measure of how well the heart is contracting, and the left ventricular (LV) wall. Exercise is started at a slower "warm-up" speed. The speed of the treadmill and its slope or inclination is increased every 3 minutes. The treadmill is abruptly stopped when the patient exceeds 85% of their target heart rate (based on the patient's age).

  Exercise may be stopped early if the patient develops signs and symptoms. Immediately after stopping the treadmill, patients move directly to the examination table and lies on their left side. The echo examination is immediately repeated. Images are stored and then played back by the computer. A video clip of multiple views of the resting and exercise study are compared side-by-side. Normal cardiac response to an increase in heart rate is an increased EF. Also, the LV walls should not demonstrate any exercise-induced abnormal movement. In contrast, a drop in EF and/or a new wall motion abnormality is an indicator of disease.

- Dobutamine Stress Echocardiography: A resting study is completed, which provides a baseline examination and demonstrates the size and function of various chambers of the heart. Focus is on the patient's resting ejection fraction (EF), a measure of how well the heart is contracting, and the left ventricular wall. Used when a physician wants to assess the heart muscle under stress.

  If exercise on a treadmill is not an option, due to a person's medical condition, a physician may use an intravenous medication called dobutamine. Dobutamine causes the heart to beat faster and will mimic the effects of exercise on the heart. Once a particular heart rate is achieved, stress echocardiography images are obtained for comparison. The patient is closely monitored for adverse effects while the effects of the medication subside.

5. **Cardiac Catheterization**: A procedure used to diagnose and treat cardiovascular conditions. During this invasive procedure, a long thin tube called a catheter is inserted in an artery or vein in the groin, neck, or arm and then threaded through the blood vessels to the heart. The test is completed for the following diagnostic purposes :

   - Locate narrowing or blockages in the coronary arteries.
   - Perform hemodynamic assessment.
   - Evaluate cardiac pressures.
   - Biopsies.
   - Diagnose congenital heart defects.
   - Diagnose heart valve anomalies and defects.

Revascularization Procedures

Percutaneous Transluminal Coronary Angioplasty (PTCA): A catheter with a deflated balloon is inserted through the groin and "threaded" in to the narrow portion of the coronary artery. The balloon is then inflated, causing the plaque build-up to be decreased, increasing the inner diameter of the artery. This procedure can be used during active ischemia to decrease myocardial wall damage. Is usually reserved for younger individuals, those with single-vessel disease, and those with more distal sites with stenosis. Has a re-stenosis rate of 30 - 50% in 6 months versus more advanced procedures.

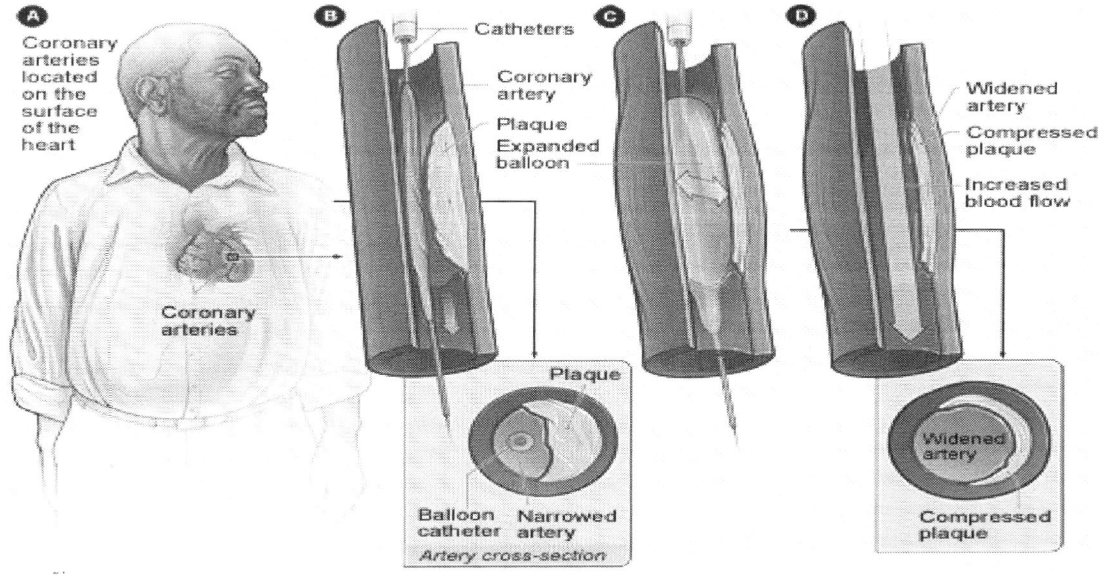

A Percutaneous Transluminal Coronary Angioplasty.

[24] Image from National Heart and Lung Institute online: http://www.nhlbi.nih.gov/health/health-topics/topics/angioplasty/howdone.html

Percutaneous Transluminal Coronary Angioplasty with Stent(s): A stent is a mesh or metal tube that acts to hold the walls of the artery open after a PTCA is performed. The stent is placed on the tip of the balloon catheter and is implanted in the artery once the blockage site is expanded. The re-stenosis rate is much lower than with traditional PTCA, about 10-15% in 6 months. Due to this, a PTCA without stent placement is becoming more obsolete. Drug-eluting stents (DES), with an immunosuppressant coating, have shown an even lower re-stenosis rate of < 5%.

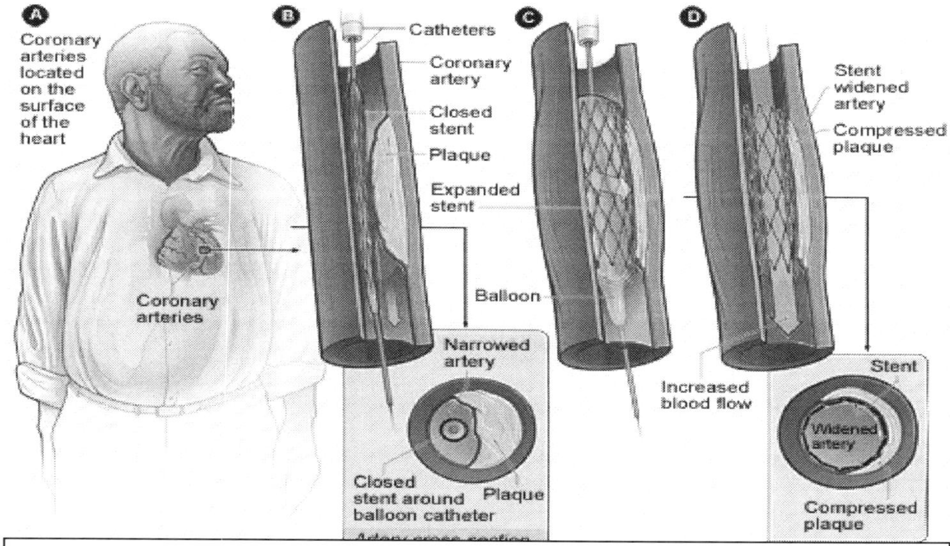

[25]

A Percutaneous Transluminal Coronary Angioplasty with Stent(s).

Laser Angioplasty: Similar in procedure to PTCA, but this is beneficial when the blockage cannot be passed through due to size and calcification of the blockage. End of the catheter emits a laser beam that breaks apart the plaque build-up. Is often used with stent placement due to the similar outcomes.

[25] Image from the National Heart and Lung Institute online: http://www.nhlbi.nih.gov/health/health-topics/topics/angioplasty/howdone.html

Coronary Artery Bypass Grafting (CABG): This procedure is indicated for those with extensive multivessel disease, who have had failed PTCA procedures, are medication resistant, or are at a high risk for future disease development. A right or left mammary artery (RIMA or LIMA), or savenous vein, is harvested and attached to the base of the aorta, below the blockage in the corresponding artery or arteries. Outcomes have shown that arterial and LIMA grafts are more resistant than savenous vein grafts (SVG) in terms of patency over a 10 year follow-up.

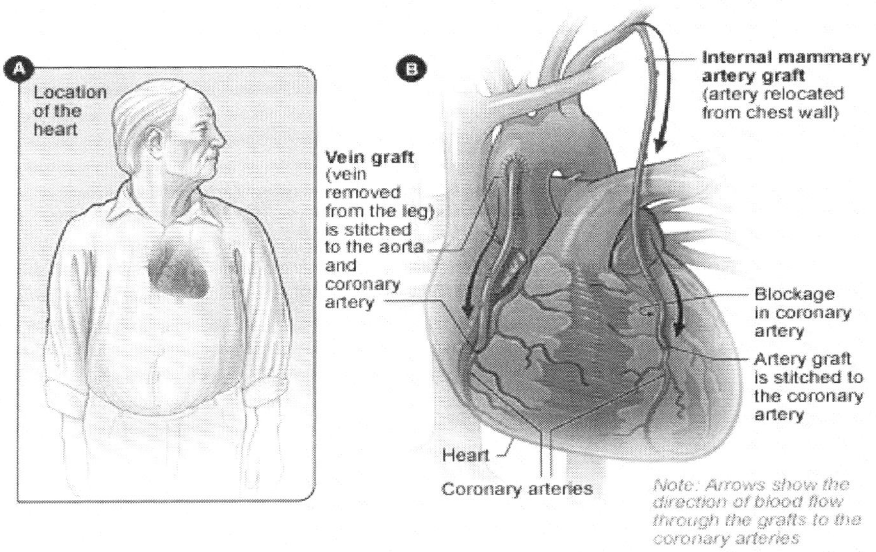

[26]

Coronary Artery Bypass Grafting.

[26] Image from the National Heart and Lung Institute online: http://www.nhlbi.nih.gov/health/health-topics/topics/cabg/

Patient Management and Medications

According to the American College of Sports Medicine (ACSM) and the American Council on Exercise (ACE), a majority of adults take one or more medications. They recognize that, while these drugs may be necessary or providing benefits, there are also side effects that impact one's ability to exercise, so it is important to know and understand the common drugs used for the management of common chronic diseases.

Antianginals
These classes of medications can cause depression, fatigue, and dizziness. Since heart rate and blood pressure is lowered, these measures are not good indicators of exercise intensity for people taking this type of medication. ACE and ACSM recommend using the Rating of Perceived Exertion (RPE) scale to monitor intensity during diagnostic testing and exercise.

1. **Beta Adrenergic Blockers**: Used to treat hypertension, left ventricular dysfunction, and angina, Beta Adrenergic Blockers Reduce ischemia by decreasing oxygen demand. These control ventricular dysrhythmias and reduce resting and exercise heart rates and blood pressures, but may increase exercise tolerance in those with ventricular dysfunction. Examples: *Toprol, Tenormin, Corgard, Inderal.*

2. **Nitrates**: Used to treat angina and as a vasodilator in heart failure, nitrates act to reduce ischemia by decreasing oxygen demand and by allowing a small increase in oxygen supply. Available in short and long lasting doses, nitrates decrease resting and exercising blood pressures. Examples: *Imdur, Nitrostat, Nitroquick, Nitrobid.*

Antihypertensives
Some individuals taking antihypertensives may experience "postural hypotension," a condition that causes a drop in systolic and/or diastolic blood pressure; leading to dizziness, light-headedness, or a loss of consciousness that could result in a fall. This occurs more frequently in those also taking diuretics. Proper hydration can play a key role in preventing this condition.

Diuretics can also cause weakness and fatigue by lowering potassium levels, a condition known as **hypokalemia**. If levels fall low enough, the risk of potentially lethal arrhythmias (VT and VF) can occur at rest or with exercise.

1. Angiotensin-Converting Enzyme (ACE) inhibitors: Used to treat hypertension, ACE inhibitors reduce myocardial oxygen demand by reducing vascular resistance and resting and exercising blood pressures; but they may increase exercise tolerance in those with left ventricular dysfunction. Examples: *Atacand, Avapro, Cozaar, Micardis, Diovan, Benicar.*

2. Calcium Channel Antagonists: Used to treat hypertension, angina, atrial fibrillation, and supraventricular tachycardia, Calcium Channel Antagonists reduce ischemia by altering the determinants of oxygen supply and demand, as well as resting and exercise blood pressures. Some may reduce resting and exercise heart rates. Examples: *Cardizem, Calan, Calan SR, Covera HS, Verelan PM.*

3. Diuretics: Used in mild hypertension, diuretics reduce blood pressure by increasing renal secretion of sodium and potassium, resulting in a loss of water in the urine, while mildly affecting resting and exercising blood pressures. These may in increase exercise tolerance in patients with congestive heart failure. There are several types:
    - Thiazides: *Hydrochlorothiazide, Indapamide.*
    - Loop: *Bumex, Lasix.*
    - Potassium-sparing: *Midamor.*
    - Aldosterone receptor blockers: *Inspra, Aldactone.*
    - Combination diuretics: *Moduretic, Maxzide.*

Antiarrhythmics

These medications can cause dizziness, dry mouth, and low blood sugar. Therefore, fluid intake and blood sugar checks should be performed on a routine basis. Exercise levels and intensities may need to be modified when appropriate.

1. **Digitalis**: Used to treat congestive heart failure, Digitalis enhances myocardial contractility, increasing stroke volume. These blunt SA and AV node conduction, reducing resting and exercise heart rates in those with tachycardia and atrial fibrillation. Digitalis, Digoxin, Lanoxin.

2. **Amiodarone**: Used to treat ventricular tachycardia, ventricular fibrillation, and atrial fibrillation, Amiodarone shows beta blocker-like and potassium channel blocker-like actions on the SA and AV nodes and increases the refractory period via sodium- and potassium-channel effects, slowing intra-cardiac conduction.

3. **Adenosine**: Used to treat supraventricular tachycardia, AV reentrant tachycardia, and AV nodal reentrant tachycardia, Adenosine causes transient heart block in the atrioventricular (AV) node. This is mediated via the A_1 receptor, inhibiting adenylyl cyclase, reducing cAMP and so causing cell hyperpolarization by increasing outward K+ flux. When Adenosine is used to cardiovert an abnormal rhythm, it is normal for the heart to enter ventricular asystole for a few seconds.

4. **Lidocaine**: Used in the treatment of stable, monomorphic, ventricular tachycardia, Lidocaine attenuates diastolic depolarization and decreases automaticity. Action potential duration and effective refractory period of ventricular muscle are decreased, raising the ventricular fibrillation threshold.

5. **Procainamide**: Used to treat supraventricular and ventricular arrhythmias, Procainamide is a sodium channel blocker which blocks open sodium channels and prolongs the cardiac action potential (outward potassium (K^+) currents may be blocked) and results in slowed conduction and, ultimately, the decreased rate of rise in the action potential.

6. **Atropine**: Used in the treatment of bradycardia, second-degree heart block Mobitz Type 1 (Wenckebach block), and third-degree heart block with a high Purkinje or AV-nodal escape rhythm, Atropine increases firing of the sinoatrial node (SA) and conduction through the atrioventricular node (AV) of the heart and blocks the action of the vagus nerve, a part of the parasympathetic system of the heart whose main action is to decrease heart rate.

Bronchodilators
Individuals with asthma or COPD may have difficulty exercising for extended durations; short, intermittent bouts of exercise may be more effective. Rests should occur as often as needed, and such individuals should begin exercise at a very low intensity. Monitor for dyspnea during the initial stages, adjusting levels appropriately. Once conditioning levels improve, gradually increase the intensity as long as the individual remain asymptomatic. It is crucial that asthma medications are taken prior to exercise and rescue inhalers are always readily available. Frequently checking Sa O2 levels with a pulse oximeter is highly recommended to help monitor exercise intensity and possible endpoints.

1. **Anticholinergics**: Used to increase the exercise capacity in patients limited by bronchospasm, Anticholingerics block the neurotransmitter acetylcholine in the central and the peripheral nervous system, affecting the muscles around the bronchi (large airways). When the lungs are irritated, these bands of muscle can tighten, narrowing the bronchi; and Anticholinergics work by stopping these muscles from tightening. Anticholinergics can increase or have no effect on resting or exercise heart rates and do not affect resting or exercising blood pressures. Examples: *Atrovent, Oxivent, Spiriva.*

2. **Sympathomimetics (Beta2-Receptor Agonists)**: These mimic the effects of transmitter substances of the sympathetic nervous system, such as catecholamines, epinephrine (adrenaline), norepinephrine (noradrenaline), and dopamine, to stimulate beta-2 receptors on the smooth muscle cells that line the airways, causing these muscle cells to relax and thereby opening airways. Sympathomimetics can increase, decrease, or have no effect on resting or exercising heart rates and blood pressures. Examples: *Serevent, Albuterol, Advair.*

3. **Anticholinergics with Sympathomimetics (Beta2-Receptor Agonists)**: These can produce a slight increase in resting and exercising heart rates and blood pressures. Examples: *Combivent, Caffeine, Theobromine*

4. **Xanthine Derivatives**: Xanthine Derivatives stimulate the central nervous system, produce diuresis, and relax smooth muscles, causing inhibition of tissue phosphodiesterases, which increases cellular cyclic AMP levels by inhibition of its breakdown and metabolism. Xanthines are also adenosine receptor antagonists, and both of these actions may be important in their effects of bronchial tree, resulting in relaxation of smooth muscle. May result in increases in the occurrence of premature ventricular contractions at rest and with exercise and in resting and exercising heart rates and blood pressures. Examples: *Caffeine, Theobromine, Theophylline, Aminophylline.*

5. **Leukotriene Antagonists and Formation Inhibitors (American Association of Family Physicians)**: Leukotrienes are potent inflammatory mediators that promote neutrophil-endothelial interactions, inducing bronchoconstriction and enhancing airway hyperresponsiveness. They also stimulate smooth muscle hypertrophy, mucus hypersecretion, and the influx of eosinophils into airway tissues. Essentially, they act by blocking 5-lipoxygenase activity. Examples: *Accolate, Singulair, Zyflo.*

6. **Mast Cell Stabilizers**: Used to prevent or control certain allergic disorders, these block a calcium channel essential for mast cell degranulation, stabilizing the cell and preventing the release of histamine and related mediators. They are used as inhalers to treat asthma, as nasal sprays to treat hay fever (allergic rhinitis), and as eye drops for allergic conjunctivitis. Examples: *Intal, Xolair.*

Antidiabetic Agents
Those with diabetes (if on insulin) must coordinate their insulin injections and food intake with their exercise program or diagnostic test. Major concerns include foot ulcers (due to peripheral vessel deterioration) and hypoglycemia (low blood sugar). The intensity, frequency, and duration of exercise will need to depend on the severity of the diabetes and an individual's overall fitness level. Those with diabetes should routinely check their blood glucose levels before and after exercise to help monitor adjustments to their intensity levels and to help avoid dangerously low blood sugar levels.

1. **Biguanides**: Decrease hepatic glucose production and intestinal glucose absorption, without effect on resting or exercising heart rates and blood pressures. Examples: *Metformin(Glucophage), Metformin/Glyburide (Glucovance).*

2. **Glucosidase Inhibitors**: These inhibit intestinal glucose absorption, and they have no effect on resting or exercising heart rates and blood pressures. Examples: *Miglitol (Glyset).*

3. **Meglitinides**: These stimulate pancreatic islet beta cells, with no effect on resting or exercising heart rates and blood pressures. Examples: *Nateglinide (Starlix), Repaglinide (Prandin).*

4. **Sulfonylureas**: These stimulate pancreatic islet beta cells, with no effect on resting or exercising heart rates and blood pressures. Examples: *Glyburide (Glynase), Glipizide (Glucotrol), Glimepiride(Amaryl).*

5. **Thiazolidinediones**: Thiazolidinediones increase insulin sensitivity, with no effect on resting or exercising heart rates and blood pressures. Examples: *Pioglitazone (Actos), Rosiglitazone (Avandia).*

6. **Insulin**: Insulin varies in how it acts, based on the type of insulin used, but it has no effect on resting or exercising heart rates and blood pressures.

   - Rapid-acting insulin is often called *mealtime insulin*, because its action curve most closely resembles the body's normal release of insulin at mealtimes. Rapid-acting insulin has an onset occurring in 5 – 15 minutes, a peak in 45 – 90 minutes, and an overall duration of about 3 – 4 hours. Examples: *Humalog, Humulin R, Novolin.*

   - Intermediate-acting insulin covers insulin needs for about half the day or overnight. This type of insulin is often combined with rapid- or short-acting insulin. It has an onset occurring in 1 – 2.5 hours, a peak in 3 – 12 hours, and an overall duration of about 18 – 24 hours. Examples: *Humulin L, Humulin N, Novolin.*

   - Long-acting insulin covers insulin needs for about one full day. This type of insulin is often combined, when needed, with rapid- or intermediate-acting insulin and has an onset occurring in 30 minutes – 3 hours, a peak onset of 6 – 20 hours, and an overall duration of 24 – 36 hours. Examples: *Humulin U, Lantus.*

Psychotropics
These medications are used to help with depression and anxiety, but can also increase drowsiness and dizziness, making it difficult to exercise. Recommendations from ACE include not exercising too soon after ingestion, ensuring that fluid intake is adequate, and ensuring that exercise durations and intensities are adjusted accordingly.

1. **Monoamine Oxidase Inhibitors (MAOIs)**: These inhibit the activity of monoamine oxidase, thus preventing the breakdown of monoamine neurotransmitters and increasing their availability. They have a long history of use as prescribed treatments for depression, but are a last choice treatment option, because they require diet restrictions since they can cause dangerously high blood pressure when taken with certain foods. Examples: *Marplan, Nardil, Emsam, Parnate.*

2. **Tricyclic Antidepressants (TCAs)**: The majority of the TCAs act primarily as serotonin-norepinephrine reuptake inhibitors (SNRIs) by blocking the serotonin transporter (SERT) and the norepinephrine transporter (NET), respectively, which results in an elevation of the synaptic concentrations of these neurotransmitters and an enhancement of neurotransmission. They are used to treat major depressive disorders, generalized anxiety disorders, obsessive compulsive disorder, and post-traumatic stress disorder and have a significantly high rate of serious cardiovascular side effects and toxicity in patients with and without known cardiovascular disease. Side effects include, but are not limited to: tachycardia, increased blood pressure, and slight prolongation of the intraventricular conduction time (leading to an increased risk of arrhythmias). They may behave as class 1A antiarrhythmics by reducing intraventricular conduction velocity and increasing collateral blood circulation or demonstrate right or left bundle branch blocks or 1st, 2nd, or 3rd degree AV heart block. Examples: *Elavil, Anafranil, Evadyne, Novaril.*

3. **Selective Serotonin Reuptake Inhibitors (SSRIs)**: Used as antidepressants in the treatment of depression, anxiety disorders, and some personality disorders, these increase the extracellular level of the neurotransmitter serotonin by inhibiting its reuptake into the presynaptic cell, increasing the level of serotonin. SSRIs have a lower side effect profile and reduced toxicity after overdose, though side effects include, but are not limited to: mild bradycardia, orthostatic hypotension, and prolongation in intraventricular conduction time, and may demonstrate QRS lengthening or prolonged QT intervals. Examples: *Celexa, Lexapro, Prozac, Paxil, Zoloft.*

Vasodilators
As most vasodilators are used in the treatment of recurrent angina, ACE recommends that those with coronary artery disease reduce physical exertion if symptoms become present, avoid exposure to extreme heat or cold, reduce emotional stress, and avoid large meals prior to exercise. Patients being treated with vasodilators run a higher risk of experiencing hypotensive episodes with postural changes and with exercise, so using the RPE scale to monitor exercise intensity is recommended.

1. **Nitrates and Nitroglycerin**: Agents that widen the blood vessels, causing a decrease in vascular resistance and an increase in blood flow. These may cause activation of the vasomotor center in the brain, which brings about relaxation of the smooth muscle in the blood vessel walls, or may act locally on blood vessel smooth muscle cells, and they can decrease resting and exercising blood pressures. Examples: *Amyl Nitrite, Imdur, NitroStat, NitroQuick, Nitro-Bid.*

2. **Direct Peripheral Vasodilators**: These medications treat hypertensive crisis, used in acute congestive heart failure, and decrease systemic blood pressure by decreasing systemic vascular resistance (arterial vasodilators) or by decreasing systemic venous return and cardiac output (venous return). They produce controlled hypotension and can decrease resting and exercising blood pressures. Examples: *Apresoline, Loniten.*

Tranquilizers
There are two main categories for tranquilizers, major and minor, which are used to induce a tranquil or relaxed state. Those taking tranquilizers are at an increased risk for drowsiness, dizziness, perspiration, and dry mouth. They are also at a greater risk for falls and complications of dehydration, so they must be monitored closely; exercise duration and intensity must be adjusted accordingly on a regular basis.

1. **Major Tranquilizers**: Widely referred to as "Neuroleptics" or "antipsychotics," these medications are used in the treatment of schizophrenia and severe paranoia disorders. Examples: *Thorazine, Haldol, Clozaril, Risperdal.*

2. **Minor Tranquilizers**: Used in the treatment of anxiety, most belong to a class known as benzodiazipenes. These can be addictive, even at prescribed dosages, if the medication is administered for long periods of time. The withdrawal process can be painful and even life-threatening, with the most common withdrawal symptoms being nausea, pain, flu-like symptoms, and seizures. Examples: *Valium, Klonopin, Ativan, Librium.*

Blood Modifiers
Patients on blood thinners must avoid vigorous exercise while they are taking these medications, as falls or injuries during vigorous exercise can cause serious internal bleeding. There are several safe forms of exercises they can engage in while taking blood thinners, including walking, swimming, and bike-riding. If a fall or injury does occur, patients need to seek immediate medical attention.

1. **Anticoagulants**: Commonly used to prevent the blood from forming dangerous clots that could result in a stroke, these are also frequently used to prevent clot formation in those with atrial fibrillation. Anticoagulants lengthen the time required to form blood clots and have no effect on resting and exercising heart rates or blood pressures. Examples: *Warfarin, Heparin.*

2. **Antiplatelets**: Frequently used after angioplasty with stent placement and valve replacement surgery, antiplatelets decrease platelet aggregation and inhibiting thrombus formation within the arterial circulation, lengthening the time it takes to form a blood clot. They have no effect on resting and exercising blood pressures when used in therapeutic doses. Examples: *Aspirin, Plavix, Aggrenox, Persantine, Ticlid.*

Caffeine
Caffeine is the most widely used stimulant. It is found in a variety of plants, dietary sources (coffee, tea, chocolate, colas), and non-prescription medications. Ingested caffeine is quickly absorbed from the stomach and peaks in the blood within 1 to 2 hours. This stimulant crosses the membranes of all tissues and has the following physiological effects:

- Increased heart rate.

- Increased blood pressure.

- Slowed breakdown of muscle glycogen and increased amount of free fatty acids in the blood stream, which enhances exercise endurance.

- Reduced amount of adenosine in the muscles, which allows an increase in muscular contractions.

- Enhanced mood, alertness, and fine motor coordination.

Nicotine
A common stimulant that has been shown to have a "biphasic effect," nicotine causes increased energy while stimulating relaxation. The most common and expedient way to get nicotine and other drugs into your bloodstream is through inhalation because the lungs are lined with millions of alveoli, the tiny air sacs where gas exchange occurs, which provide an enormous surface area and, therefore, ample access to the bloodstream.

Once in your bloodstream, nicotine flows almost immediately to the brain. Although nicotine causes many different actions throughout the body, its effect on the brain is responsible for both the positive feelings experienced during smoking and the irritability experienced during the quitting process. Nicotine does not stay in the body for long; it has a half-life of about 60 minutes, meaning that six hours after a cigarette, only about 0.031mg of the 1 mg of nicotine inhaled remains in the body. Nicotine initially causes a rapid release of adrenaline which will lead to:

- Increased heart rate and blood pressure.

- Increased respiratory rates.

- Increased muscular endurance due to higher blood sugar levels.

- Increased of arrhythmias at rest and with exercise.

While some studies have shown that consuming nicotine prior to exercise increases endurance, the long-term negative impacts of nicotine outweigh any short-term benefits.

Alcohol
Alcohol in one's system before or after exercising can have several negative effects, including but not limited to:

- Slower Recovery Time. Maximal workouts drain glycogen stores and leave your muscle tissue in need of repair. Alcohol stalls the recovery process. High levels of alcohol displace the carbohydrates, leaving stores 50% lower than normal, even after eight hours.

- Increasing Body Fat Percentage. When alcohol is present, the body – besides having to deal with the surplus of calories – prioritizes metabolizing the alcohol over burning fat and carbohydrates. Alcohol also breaks down amino acids and stores them as fat, especially in the thighs and gluteals. Excessive alcohol consumption can significantly deteriorate muscles in those areas and increase levels of cortisol (a stress hormone), which further encourages fat storage, particularly in the midsection.

- Disrupted Sleep. Excessive alcohol intake decreases muscle recovery and performance by disrupting sleep. Alcohol decreases sleep duration and increases wakefulness (particularly in the second half of the night), especially in women. Disrupting the sleep cycle can reduce human growth hormone output – which builds muscle – by as much as 70%.

- Depletion of Water and Nutrients. Alcohol irritates the stomach lining, which can reduce your capacity to absorb nutrients and acts as a diuretic. For every gram of ethanol you drink, you excrete out 10 milliliters of urine, the equivalent of about 9.5 ounces of urine for two beers, which can cause dehydration; as little as 2% dehydration hurts endurance performance.

Diet Pills

These products achieve their effects in several ways, most unsafe; *Ephedrine* and *Country Mallow* have already been banned by the FDA. They affect the body in the following ways:

- Blocking or decreasing the amount of fat absorbed from the food, as in drugs such as *Alli, Chitosan,* and *Guar Gum.*

- Decreasing your appetite, such as with *Ephedra, Hoodia,* and *Country Mallow.*

- Increasing the amount of calories individuals burn, including *Bitter Orange*, *Chromium*, and green tea extract.

Long-term use of diet pills can have serious consequences. Taking diet pills results in higher likelihood of **primary pulmonary hypertension**, a disease that increases pressure on the arteries in your lungs, breathing problems, often followed by the need for a lung transplant, heart palpitations, stroke, and increased blood pressure.

Antihistamines

When the body is affected by an outside substance, like pollen, it reacts by producing histamines, which are the body's defense against these invaders. Unfortunately, in defensively creating histamines, it also creates the symptoms that come with them, such as watery eyes, sneezing, coughing, and, in extreme cases, shortness of breath and asthma. Antihistamines reduce the effects of our body's defense mechanism. Common side effects of antihistamines are:

- Drowsiness.

- Dizziness and blurred vision.

- Restlessness and nervousness.

- Upset stomach.

- Dry mouth, dry nose.

- Irritability.

- Difficulty urinating.

Antihistamines do not have any proven negative effects on physical activities, though the side effects of the drugs are not always pleasant. The fatigue that can result from taking some antihistamines, along with the dry of mouth and nasal passages, may make concentration during workouts more difficult. Staying hydrated throughout the exercise session may improve dry nose and mouth symptoms and timing allergy medication use to not coincide with physical activity, if possible, may help individuals feel more energetic.

An individual who feels lightheaded, dizzy, or faint after a workout could be suffering from low blood pressure associated with exercise. Post-exercise fainting can be reduced or prevented in some cases with antihistamine drugs that are usually prescribed to treat seasonal allergies and acid reflux.

Cold Medications

Many common over-the-counter cold medications can cause side effects if you exercise. While most people know that the caffeine is found in coffee and colas, many don't realize that cold medications also may contain compounds that can elevate the heart rate.

For most people, taking any one of these in a normal dose probably wouldn't cause a problem, but with the addition of exercise (also a stimulant) one may experience unwanted side effects. These include, but are not limited to:

- Increased resting and exercising heart rates and blood pressures.
- Increased atrial and/or ventricular ectopic beats.
- Irritability and anxiety.

Some drugs may hurt exercise performance by impairing coordination and judgment, causing drowsiness or accelerating dehydration. Others, due to their stimulant properties, may enhance performance, though often with risk.

Test Your Knowledge: Medical and Surgical Management

1. True/False: In terms of chronological age, adolescence ranges from the ages of mid 20's to late 40's.

2. Name four physiological considerations when designing exercise prescriptions for children.

3. True/False: State anxiety, trait anxiety, and burn-out are three psychological considerations to keep in mind when encouraging routine exercise for children.

4. What is a benefit of exercise in older age groups (65 and older)?
   a) Improved psychological and cognitive well-being.
   b) An increase in chronic disease states.
   c) Reduction in physical injuries/impairments.
   d) Both a) and c).
   e) All of the above.

5. What type of test measures how well the lungs are oxygenating blood in patients being assessed for COPD?
   a) Chest X-ray.
   b) Pulmonary Function Test.
   c) Arterial Blood Gas Analysis.
   d) CT scan.

6. True/False: Sarcoidosis is an example of a restrictive lung disease extrinsic in origin.

7. Which of the following is a non-modifiable risk factor for CVD?
   a) Smoking.
   b) Gender.
   c) Hypertension.
   d) Dyslipidemia.
   e) Type II diabetes.

8. Which medication is used in the treatment of mild hypertension?
   a) Calcium Channel Blockers.
   b) Nitrates.
   c) Beta Blockers.
   d) Diuretics.

9. List five signs and symptoms of Cardiopulmonary Disease.

10. True/False: The American Heart Association describes insulin resistance as when the body cannot properly use insulin or glucose with a fasting blood glucose level greater than or equal to120mg/dL.

11. The effects of exercise on coronary artery disease risk factors are:
    a) A decrease in resting and exercise blood pressure.
    b) A decrease in total cholesterol, LDL cholesterol, and triglycerides.
    c) An increase in HDL cholesterol.
    d) Improved glucose tolerance and insulin sensitivity.
    e) All of the above.

12. True/False: Calcium channel antagonists are used to treat high blood pressure, angina, atrial fibrillation, and supraventricular tachycardia.

13. List four characteristics of transmural ischemia with myocardial infarction.

14. The following are steps to assist in behavior adherence:
  a) Assess the individual's medical needs.
  b) Identify specific medication goals.
  c) Plan the teaching-learning and behavioral change process.
  d) Establish support.
  e) All of the above

15. True/False: Stress echocardiography involves the use of a radioactive tracer to assess blood flow to the myocardium at rest and after peak exercise.

16. Name 3 types (classes) of antianginals.

17. Which is an example of an antianginal medication?
  a) Toprol.
  b) Nitroquick.
  c) Lasix.
  d) Both a) and b).
  e) None of the above.

18. Which is a side effect of diuretics?
  a) Tachycardia.
  b) Headaches.
  c) Postural Hypotension.
  d) Blurred vision.

19. List 3 characteristics of amiodarone.

20. What are the 3 types of insulin used in diabetes management?

21. Which of the following is/are side effect(s) of Tricyclic antidepressants (TCA's)?
  a) Bradycardia.
  b) Hypertension.
  c) Left and/or Right Bundle Branch Blocks on ECG.
  d) Both b) and c).
  e) All of the above.

22. True/False: Selective Serotonin Reuptake Inhibitors (SSRI's) have a high side effect profile and reduced toxicity after overdose.

23. Name 5 kinds of anti-platelet medications.

24. Please list the 4 reasons why alcohol consumption and exercise is contraindicated.

25. True/False: Taking an antihistamine prior to exercise is recommended to boost energy levels.

Test Your Knowledge: Medical and Surgical Management – Answers

1. **False.** Adolescence ranges from 16 years to early 20s.

2. The following are all correct answers:
    - Higher maximal and submaximal oxygen uptake.
    - Higher resting and exercising heart rates.
    - Lower resting and exercising blood pressures.
    - Hormonal changes.
    - Thermoregulatory differences.
    - Muscle and bone formation.
    - Body composition.

3. **True.**

4. **d)** Both **a)** and **c)** are benefits.

5. **c)** Arterial Blood Gas Analysis.

6. **False.** It is an example of an intrinsic RLD).

7. **b)** Gender.

8. **d)** Diuretics.

9. The following are all correct answers:
    - Pain or discomfort in the chest, neck, jaw, or back.
    - Resting dyspnea or dizziness.
    - Nocturnal dyspnea.
    - Orthopnea.
    - Ankle edema.
    - Palpitations.
    - Claudications.
    - Heart Murmurs.
    - Unusual fatigue.

10. **False.** Level is < or equal to 110mg/dL.

11. **b)** All of the above.

12. **True.**

13. Any of the following are correct:
    - Changes in both QRS and ST complexes.
    - ST elevation or Tall, upright T-waves early on.
    - Q waves in a few hours after onset.
    - ST elevation may return to baseline and T wave invert.
    - Q waves may persist for years; T wave inversion may indefinitely.

14. c) Plan the teaching-learning and behavioral change process.

15. False.

16. Beta Adrenergic Blockers, Nitrates, Calcium Channel Antagonists.

17. d) Both a) and b).

18. c) Postural Hypotension.

19. Used to treat ventricular tachycardia, ventricular fibrillation, and atrial fibrillation; Shows beta blocker-like and Potassium channel blocker-like actions on the SA and AV node; Increases the refractory period via sodium and potassium channel effects which slow intracardiac conduction.

20. Rapid, Intermediate, and Long-acting insulin are all used in diabetes management.

21. d) Both b) and c).

22. False. A lower side effect profile with a reduced toxicity after overdose.

23. Aspirin, Plavix, Persantine, Aggrenox, Ticlid.

24. Decreased recovery time, increase in body fat percentage, disrupted sleep, and depletion of water and nutrients.

25. False. Avoid taking an antihistamine prior to exercise to help avoid fatigue during session.

Chapter 11: Pathophysiology and Risk Factors

Pathophysiology can be defined simply as the study of biological function during states of disease. **Risk factors** describe variables associated with the different types of diseases within the body. An understanding of pathophysiology and risk factors is critical for a health fitness professional, especially one looking to create a successful exercise program.

Exercise and Those with Chronic Diseases

There are a variety of common chronic diseases which impact the health of individuals interested in pursuing a fitness regimen. Physiological and metabolic responses to exercise are frequently heavily influenced by specific disease conditions. Some of the most common chronic diseases requiring identification and understanding by certified personal trainers include the following:

Hypertension

Hypertension, or high blood pressure, is a chronic medical condition in which the blood pressure in the arteries is elevated. The American Heart Association guidelines indicate that normal blood pressure readings for an adult over the age of 20 should be less than 120/80 mm Hg. Blood pressures are subject to change rapidly – depending upon factors such as posture, sleep, stress, or exercise – so this is meant to be a general guideline. The American Heart Association reports that approximately one out of three American adults suffers from hypertension.

Exercise and Hypertension
Blood pressure is determined by the amount of blood the heart pumps, coupled with the level of resistance to blood flow in the arteries. Narrowed arteries result in high blood pressure and can lead to life-threatening illnesses such as heart attacks and strokes. Exercise increases the flow of blood throughout the body. Therefore, the presence of narrowed arteries makes increased physical activity a concern for individuals with uncontrolled hypertension because it can result in the heart struggling to supply the brain and body with blood that carries critical oxygen.

High blood pressure can lead to a **hypertensive crisis**, which is classified as blood pressure over 180/110. These blood pressure readings are considered a medical emergency. On the other hand, it is possible for an individual to suffer from hypertension for long periods of time without any symptoms.

Risk Factors
Hypertension
Blood pressure should be under control and well-maintained prior to beginning an exercise regimen. As few symptoms are associated with high blood pressure, it's often referred to as "the silent killer." Individuals taking blood pressure-lowering medications known as **diuretics** need to be especially vigilant about the possibility of dehydration. Diuretics are used to increase urination, which decreases the amount of fluids flowing throughout blood vessels. This process ultimately lowers the pressure of fluid pushing against vessels of the body. However, increased urination also puts an individual at risk for dehydration. Adequate hydration during exercise is critical for individuals using diuretics to control hypertension.

Metabolic Diseases

Metabolic Syndrome refers to a group of conditions related to the body's metabolism. These conditions include excess body fat, elevated triglycerides, blood pressure, and blood sugar, and low HDL cholesterol. Risk factors that may require a medical consultation prior to testing or training include:

Obesity
An adult who has a BMI of 30 or higher is considered obese. Another standard that defines obesity is a weight more than 20% above the recommended norm for one's age, sex, and height. Exercise can actually be dangerous to the cardiovascular health of severely overweight individuals. They are also at a greater risk for physical injury.

Thyroid Disease
When the thyroid malfunctions, hormone levels, metabolism, energy and weight can fluctuate. Low energy levels and muscle weakness are common problems linked with thyroid disorders. These symptoms can affect an individual's ability to tolerate exercise.

Diabetes Mellitus
As mentioned in previous chapters, diabetes occurs as a result of either inadequate insulin production or the inability of the body's cells to respond properly to insulin. Sometimes a diagnosis of diabetes can be related to both of these factors. There are three classifications of diabetes mellitus: Type I, Type II, and gestational diabetes.

Exercise is important for people with diabetes because it helps control blood sugar levels and assists with the management of body weight. However, care should be taken when planning and implementing exercise programs for persons affected by diabetes because **hypoglycemia** (low blood sugar) or **hyperglycemia** (high blood sugar) can occur as a result of exercise.

The most common signs and symptoms of **hypoglycemia** include: shakiness, dizziness, sweating, hunger, headache, confusion, and behavioral changes

The most frequent signs and symptoms of **hyperglycemia** include: high blood glucose, increased urination, and increased thirst.

The American Diabetes Association outlines the following target blood sugar levels for the majority of diabetics who are not pregnant. However, guidelines may differ among some diabetic individuals based on their primary care physician's plan of care:

Glucose Reading Prior to a Meal: 70–130 mg/dl.
Glucose Reading Following a Meal: <180 mg/dl.

Immunosuppressive Disease
This medical condition refers to various diseases that suppress the immune system, and is sometimes called **immune deficiency**. **Primary immune deficiency** disorders involve congenital defects of the immune system. Examples include Selective IgA Deficiency, Common Variable Immunodeficiency, X-Linked Agammaglobulinemia, andChronic Granulomatous Disease.

Acquired immunodeficiency involves the acquisition of an immune deficiency due to certain diseases, rather than an individual being born with the condition. AIDS is the most widely recognized disease associated with this category. Cancer patients undergoing chemotherapy commonly develop this condition. Transplant patients who take immunosuppression medications to better accept the introduction of a new organ are a high risk group.

Exercise and Metabolic Disorders

It should be noted that individuals with an elevated blood sugar level above 240 mg/dl should avoid exercise. A diabetic client should check their urine for **ketones** – substances produced when the body breaks down fat for energy – at this point. Normally, the body gets the energy it needs from carbohydrates. However, when an individual's diet does not include enough carbohydrates, stored fats are broken down, increasing the amount of ketones in the urine. This increased presence is most common in Type I diabetes. A significant amount of ketones can poison the body.

Risk Factors

The greatest exercise risk for individuals with diabetes is hypoglycemia, the risk of which is greatest after high-intensity or long sessions of exercise. The ACSM recommends that diabetic individuals inject insulin according to their primary care physician's recommendations at least one hour prior to exercise. It's also critical for diabetic individuals to ensure adequate food intake.

A diabetic needs to monitor his or her blood-glucose levels before and after engaging in a fitness workout. Close monitoring is also recommended when engaging in a new type of activity or exercise. Diabetics should keep a source of fast-acting carbohydrates with them while exercising and also inform other individuals where the emergency source is located in case hypoglycemia occurs.

Pulmonary Disease

Pulmonary disease refers to disorders related to the lungs and respiratory system. Chronic obstructive pulmonary disease (**COPD**) is one of the most common types of pulmonary disease, frequently involving a diagnosis of both emphysema and chronic bronchitis.

Emphysema

This disease involves damage to the air sacs within the lung, resulting in a loss of elasticity. The primary symptom of emphysema is shortness of breath upon exertion. As this disorder progresses, shortness of breath will occur with mild activities or while an individual is at rest.

Chronic Bronchitis

The hallmarks of this pulmonary disease include the presence of a chronic cough and excessive mucous production. These symptoms are related to swelling and irritation of the lungs. Smoking is a primary contributor to the conditions of emphysema and chronic bronchitis. Regular physical activity can reduce the workload on the lungs by building up endurance. Physical activity is also associated with improved quality of life, but it is critical to follow a doctor's recommendations for activity levels and restrictions.

To manage shortness of breath, individuals with pulmonary diseases can utilize **pursed lip breathing**, which, by slowing the pace of breathing, improves ventilation of the lungs and keeps the airways open longer. Pursed lip breathing is especially effective during difficult parts of physical activity.

Pursed Lip Breathing Technique

1. Relax.
2. Breathe in slowly through the nose for two counts, keeping the mouth closed.

3. Pucker or "purse" the lips (as if getting ready to whistle).

4. Breathe out slowly and gently through pursed lips while counting to four.

Asthma
Asthma is a chronic lung disease which occurs as a result of swollen and inflamed airways, leading to the obstruction of airflow through the lungs. The most common symptoms of asthma include wheezing, chest tightness, shortness of breath, and coughing.

Exercise and Pulmonary Diseases
Let's dispel a common myth. Individuals with pulmonary lung disease are NOT too short of breath to exercise. There are numerous benefits related to exercise for these individuals. A medically-appropriate exercise regimen increases energy levels, endurance, muscle strength, and bone density, while improving the ability to combat infections. It also promotes restful sleep and relaxation.

The goal of an asthma-treatment exercise plan, in particular, is to keep symptoms under control, so that asthmatic individuals can enjoy exercising. Certain activities are better suited for those with asthma, such as: swimming, walking, biking, and hiking. It's best to avoid physical activities linked with cold weather, such as cross-country skiing and ice hockey, as those tend to exacerbate symptoms related to difficult breathing.

To ensure safety during an exercise routine, asthmatic individuals can adhere to the following precautions:

- Using pre-exercise inhalers as prescribed by a medical professional prior to participating in exercise.

- Performing warm-up exercises and using appropriate cool-down periods following exercise.

- Avoiding exercise in cold temperatures. This will likely exasperate asthma symptoms and make breathing more difficult.

- Restricting exercise when a viral infection, such as a cold, is present.

- Maintaining an exercise regimen that is medically appropriate.

- An individual with pulmonary disease who experiences difficulty breathing while exercising should stop activity and repeat a pre-exercise inhaled medication. If the symptoms are relieved, exercise can continue. If the systems return, the inhaler should be repeated and a doctor should be notified for further direction.

Risk Factors
The ACSM supports light to moderate physical activity (30 minutes daily) for individuals diagnosed with pulmonary disorders such as emphysema, chronic bronchitis, and asthma. The ACSM does recommend a medically-monitored exercise evaluation prior to the beginning of a fitness program to determine if there is a need for medical support and surveillance during exercise. This assessment can also help determine the optimal training heart rate as well as an appropriate training intensity, duration, and frequency for each patient.

The following specific recommendations for exercise considerations are directly from the "Current Comment" by the ACSM on "Exercise for Persons with Chronic Obstructive Pulmonary Disease":

> *Aerobic training should involve the major muscle groups of the lower extremities, as these are used in everyday tasks such as walking and climbing stairs, for a total of 20 to 30 minutes. Improved walking endurance, activity tolerance and quality of life have been reported after programs using either stationary cycling, ground-based and treadmill walking, or a combination of all three. Since numerous daily activities require use of the upper extremities, endurance and strength training of the upper body can also provide practical benefits. It is advisable to combine resistance training with an aerobic training program to help increase endurance. Exercises for strengthening should include all major muscle groups. The resistance should be prescribed for each person and allow for completion of at least one set of 8 to 12 repetitions of the exercise. As muscular strength and endurance improve, more sets can be added to each exercise.*

Exercise-induced bronchospasm occurs when the airways in the lungs shrink during exercise, resulting in difficulty with breathing. Exercising for extended periods of time may not be tolerated by individuals with this condition.

Musculoskeletal Disorders

The musculoskeletal system of the body includes all of the muscles, bones, joints, and related structures, such as tendons and connective tissue that work together to enable the movement of the body. When any of these parts of the musculoskeletal system are not functioning properly, exercise can be difficult. Physical activity may be contraindicated in certain conditions or modifications may be necessary for safety.

Acute or Chronic Back Pain
Back pain is one of the most commonly seen medical problems. It's estimated by the National Institute of Arthritis and Musculoskeletal and Skin Diseases that eight out of ten people at some point during their lives will be affected by this condition. Acute back pain occurs suddenly and can last from a few days to a few weeks. Back pain is considered chronic if it lasts for more than three months.

Low Back Pain
The back tends to lose bone strength and muscle elasticity as individuals grow older. That lack of elasticity and strength, coupled with overstretching or overstraining the muscles, can result in sprains, strains, or spasms of the muscles of the back. Damage to the spongy cartilage between the vertebrae of the back, called intervertebral discs, sometimes results in painful bulges or ruptures of these fluid-filled "shock absorbers" within the spinal column. Pressure from these bulges or ruptures commonly affect the numerous nerves throughout the spinal cord, creating extreme low back pain.

Additional factors (beside trauma) can lead to low back pain as well. Degenerative diseases such as arthritis, osteoporosis, and viral infections are often the root cause of low back pain. Obesity, stress, smoking, and a poor level of physical fitness are also believed to contribute to this musculoskeletal disorder.

Tendonitis
Tendons connect muscle to bone. When a muscle contracts, it transmits force through the tendon and to the bone, enabling the body to walk, jump, climb, etc. **Tendonitis** refers to the irritation and inflammation of a tendon. Common symptoms include:

- Tenderness of the area over the tendon.
- Pain that occurs with the movement of muscles and tendons.
- Swelling of the tendon.

Tendinitis can occur in any tendon, but most commonly in the rotator cuff, elbow, knee, or wrist. Rest and the application of ice to the affected area are common treatments for tendonitis. Gentle exercises, once pain in the area of the tendonitis subsides, can be beneficial if a medical professional has ruled out any other musculoskeletal problems.

Osteoporosis
The National Institutes of Health reports that over 40 million people either already have osteoporosis or are at high risk for developing this bone disorder. Numerous risk factors lead to the onset of osteoporosis, a condition that results in the weakening of the bones.

Fractures of the hip, spine, and wrist are most common in those stricken by this musculoskeletal disease.

The American College of Sports Medicine Resource Manual suggests the following recommendations regarding exercise for those with a diagnosis of osteoporosis:

- One to three sets —with five to eight repetitions— of four to six weight-bearing, lower-body strength exercises using body weight as resistance
- Exercise regimens two to three times per week
- Additional resistance can be added over a period of time with weighted vests (max of 10 lbs.)
- Therapy bands are recommended in the use of range-of-motion exercises
- Impact exercise, spinal flexion against resistance, spinal extension, high compressive forces on the spine, and quick trunk rotation are activities contraindicated for individuals.

Osteoarthritis
The Arthritis Foundation reports that 27 million people in the United States are affected by osteoarthritis (OA), which is the most common type of arthritis. This disorder of the musculoskeletal system involves the breakdown of cartilage. Cartilage cushions the joints to keep bones from rubbing against one another during movement. Pain and stiffness are the primary symptoms when a breakdown of cartilage occurs. Consequently, joint replacement procedures are often required as a result of OA.

Exercise can actually help those suffering from OA by reducing joint pain, making it easier to complete everyday activities. Heat and cold therapy are effective tools for managing discomfort associated with OA following exercise. The American Orthopedic Society for Sports Medicine recommends an exercise program for those suffering from OA that involves a routine lasting between 30 and 45 minutes with a frequency of three to five times per week.

Rheumatoid Arthritis (RA)
Rheumatoid arthritis (RA) is a form of inflammatory arthritis and an autoimmune disease. Those coping with RA have an immune system that attacks their body's own tissues. Inflammation primarily affects

the lining of the joints and can lead to the break-down of cartilage and bone. Pain, swelling, and redness of the joints are frequent symptoms of RA.

Inactivity decreases joint motion and flexibility, leads to weakened muscles, and contributes to the deformity of joints. Exercise can actually reverse joint stiffness and help those coping with RA experience a decrease in fatigue and an increase in muscle tone.

The Centers for Disease Control and Prevention (CDC) recommend that those with RA aged younger than 65 – who are not limited in their regular functioning and do not suffer from the chronic conditions of diabetes, heart disease, or cancer – should follow these exercise guidelines for maximum health benefits:

> 5 hours of moderate intensity aerobic exercise, or 2 ½ hours of vigorous intensity exercise with the same amount and frequency of muscle strengthening activities per week.

Individuals over the age of 65 with limited functioning or additional chronic diseases are advised by the CDC to follow similar recommendations. In addition, integrating activities that support balance into an exercise routine at least three days per week is recommended.

Exercise and Musculoskeletal Disorders

Regular exercise helps keep back muscles strong and can be a key preventative measure against developing acute and chronic back pain. The National Institute of Neurological Disorders and Stroke contends that exercise is one of the best ways to recover from low back pain.

However, they also caution that moderate pain experienced for more than 15 minutes during exercise is an indicator that one should stop the exercise and consult with a medical professional should be sought.

Risk Factors

Musculoskeletal conditions are impacted by numerous risk factors which require consideration before prescribing an exercise routine. Some of these risk factors are modifiable. Therefore, an individual can takes steps to decrease these risk factors. Other risk factors are not modifiable.

Modifiable Risk Factors

- Sedentary lifestyle.
- Cigarette smoking.
- Inadequate physical fitness level.
- Use or lack of use of protective equipment.
- Exposure to unfavorable environmental conditions.

Non-Modifiable Risk Factors

- **Age**: The aging process results in a progressive decline in muscle mass, loss of connective tissue elasticity, and the thinning of cartilage between the joints. Soft tissue damage over the course of a lifetime takes its toll on the body. Further, the body's ability to heal slows down.
- Gender
- Prior history of injury.
- History of inadequate physical activity in the past.
- Anatomical factors.

Heart Disease

The term heart disease includes several conditions: coronary artery disease, heart rhythm problems (arrhythmias), heart infections, heart defects an individual is born with (congenital heart defects), etc.

Coronary Artery Disease

Coronary arteries supply oxygen-rich blood to the heart muscle. **Coronary artery disease** (CAD) develops when waxy substances, known as plaque, build up inside the coronary arteries: a process known as **atherosclerosis**.

Over time, plaque buildup narrows the coronary arteries and reduces the flow of blood to the heart. The plaques can rupture, leading to the formation of life-threatening blood clots. CAD can also lead to a heart attack, heart failure, and arrhythmias.

Damage to the inner layers of the coronary arteries contributes to the process of this disease and those with the following risk factors have a higher chance of incurring this damage:

- Smoking.
- High levels of certain fats and cholesterol in the blood.
- Hypertension.
- Elevated levels of sugar in the blood due to insulin resistance or diabetes.
- Blood vessel inflammation.
- Obesity.
- Lack of physical activity.
- Unhealthy diet.
- Family history of early heart disease.

Myocardial Ischemia

Myocardial ischemia occurs with decreased blood flow through one or more of the blood vessels leading to the heart. This in turn decreases the amount of oxygen reaching the heart muscle (myocardium). Myocardial ischemia may occur slowly as arteries become blocked over time, or it may occur quickly when an artery becomes blocked suddenly. This process results in tissue damage. Myocardial ischemia is commonly referred to as angina or chest pain.

Typical Angina

This type of chest pain is often called **stable angina** and is the most common. It occurs during physical activity and has a predictable pattern. Rest and/or angina medication such as nitroglycerine typically relieves this type of angina.

Atypical angina

Atypical, or **unstable angina** as it's commonly called, doesn't follow a regular pattern. It can occur while at rest or during physical activity. Rest and/or medication are not effective in relieving the discomfort associated with this angina. Immediate emergency consultation is recommended because it's a sign that a heart attack could occur at any time.

Vasospastic Angina

This medical condition involves spasms of one or both of the coronary arteries resulting in restricted blood flow to the heart. Vasospastic angina is different from a typical angina because it typically occurs while at rest. It is sometimes referred to as **Prinzmetal's angina** or **variant angina**.

Some individuals experience ischemia without feeling any chest pain, discomfort, or other symptoms. This condition is known as **silent ischemia** and is most prevalent in women, older individuals, and those with a diabetes diagnosis.

The American College of Sports Medicine (ACSM) guideline for exercise prescription in patients with ischemia/angina states:

> *Because symptomatic or silent ischemia may be arrhythmogenic, the THR (training heart rate) for endurance exercise should be set safely below (>10 beats/min) the ischemic ECG or anginal threshold. Alternately, the upper heart level can be set as the highest non ischemic workload from a Graded Exercise Tolerance (GXT).*

Myocardial Infarction

The process leading to a myocardial infarction is the same as that leading to myocardial ischemia, but it results in tissue death and is more critical. A myocardial infarction is commonly referred to as a heart attack. Additional causes of myocardial ischemia and infarction include:

Atherosclerosis

A build-up of cholesterol within the arteries, atherosclerosis causes blockages of blood flow to the heart.

Blood Clots

When plaque from atherosclerosis ruptures, it results in a blood clot, which may lead to sudden myocardial ischemia, resulting in a heart attack.

Coronary Spasms

These brief, temporary contractions of the muscles in the artery wall can lead to a decrease or even a complete blockage of blood flow to the heart.

The body heals damage to the myocardium following ischemia or infarction through the formation of scar tissue; and the healing process actually begins as soon as blood flow is restored. White blood corpuscles move into the damaged heart muscle and remove the dead cells. Gradually, scar tissue forms in the area of the heart that was damaged. The healing process typically takes four to eight weeks to complete.

Numerous complications are possible following an acute myocardial infarction, including the occurrence of an additional infarction. Other potential complications include the following:

Congestive Heart Failure

A myocardial infarction may reduce the ability of the heart to act as a pump for the circulation within the body. This condition is known as congestive heart failure. Individuals with diabetes are particularly at risk in developing this complication.

Myocardial Rupture

Myocardial rupture is a tear that occurs in the myocardium. It can also involve the small muscles that pull on the heart valves, or the flaps of the heart valves themselves. Prognosis is generally poor, and death can result from this complication, but medical intervention is sometimes effective.

Arrhythmia
Infarctions change the electrical characteristics of the tissue damaged within the heart, altering the normal rhythms of the heart.

Pericarditis
The inflammatory response from an infarction can affect the sac that lines the heart known as the **pericardium**. This condition is called pericarditis.

Cardiogenic Shock
Cardiogenic shock results when the heart is unable to produce enough of a cardiac output to supply an adequate amount of oxygenated blood to the tissues of the body. This complication is rare, but can be fatal if not treated immediately.

The American Heart Association (AHA) endorses the following diet recommendations for general heart health for children older than age two and adults with or without health problems:

- Eat a variety of fruit and vegetable servings daily.
- Eat a variety of grain products every day.
- Eat fish at least two times weekly. Oily fish, which omega-3 fatty acids, are best particularly for your heart.
- Maintain a healthy weight by balancing the amount of calories consumed with daily activity. To lose weight, increase activity level to burn more calories than are consumed.
- Eat foods low in saturated fat and cholesterol.
- Limit the amount of trans fat in the diet. These fats raise the levels of LDL cholesterol while lowering HDL cholesterol in the blood.
- Limit sodium intake to less than 2,300 mg of sodium a day.
- Limit alcohol intake to two drinks a day for men and one drink a day for women.
- Limit drinks and foods with added sugar.

Exercise and Heart Disease
Exercise builds strength in many muscles within the body, including the heart. A stronger heart lowers blood pressure responses to activity, which in turn reduces strain placed on the heart. When conditioned by exercise, the heart's capacity to pump blood throughout the body increases. In addition, the resting heart rate of an individual who participates in regular exercise is slower (because less effort is required to pump blood). With all of these effects in mind, it is obvious to see how exercise is an excellent deterrent to heart disease. It keeps the artery walls flexible, thereby lowering blood pressure; helps individuals reduce their weight, which reduces strain on the entire cardiovascular system; and improves cholesterol and fat levels are frequently observed in those who exercise regularly.

Risk Factors
Individuals with existing heart problems such as heart arrhythmias or a history of previous heart attacks should seek guidance from a medical professional prior to beginning a fitness routine. Symptoms of arrhythmias include the feeling of fluttering in the chest, rapid heart rate, or the feeling that the heart is skipping beats. The major symptoms of a heart attack are angina or chest pain.

Young adults with congenital heart defects such as hypertrophic cardiomyopathy or myocarditis should also seek medical advice about safe forms of exercise. CAD should also be stable prior to engaging in a fitness program. Symptoms of uncontrolled CAD are shortness of breath or chest discomfort.

Cardiovascular Risk Factors
Let's break down the risk factors of cardiovascular complications more clearly:

Inappropriate Changes of Resting or Exercise Heart Rate or Blood Pressure
The heart beats about 60 to 80 times a minute under normal conditions. Blood pressure rises with each heartbeat and falls when the heart relaxes between beats. Resting Heart Rate (RHR) is the rate at which the heart beats when an individual is at rest. Blood pressure is constantly subject to change, and is related to changes in posture, exercise, or sleeping. Drastic changes in resting or exercise heart rates or blood pressure should be investigated immediately.

Target heart rates while exercising are expressed as percentages of an individual's maximum heart rate that are safe and offer maximum benefits from a workout. The American Heart Association recommends an exercise target heart rate for most people ranging from 50% to 75% of an individual's maximum heart rate. This is commonly calculated as "220 minus the individual's age."

New Onset of Discomfort in Chest, Neck, Shoulder, or Arm; Changes in the Pattern of Discomfort during Rest or Exercise
This type of discomfort can be an early warning sign of a possible heart attack.

Fainting or Dizzy Spells
An individual experiencing fainting episodes or feelings of dizziness needs a medical evaluation. These are prime indicators that difficulties with blood flow may be present.

Claudication
Claudication is pain and/or cramping in the lower leg due to inadequate blood flow to the muscles. The most common cause of claudication is peripheral artery disease. This is a chronic disease that may result from atherosclerosis.

Cardiovascular System and Exercise
Exercise puts an increased demand on the cardiovascular system. Oxygen demand by the muscles rises significantly. Metabolic processes speed up and more waste is formed. Increased nutrients are used and body temperature rises. The cardiovascular system works to regulate these changes and meet the body's demands. Chronic or acute disease can compromise these normal cardiovascular system responses to exercise.

Heart Rate
The heart rate increases in direct proportion to exercise intensity until a maximum heart rate is reached. Resting heart rate can decrease significantly following training in a previously sedentary individual. Maximum heart rate tends to remain unchanged by training and is influenced by genetics. Following an exercise session, heart rate remains elevated before slowly recovering to a resting level. After a period of fitness training, the time it takes for heart rate to recover to its resting value is normally lessened.

Stroke Volume
Stroke volume is the amount of blood ejected per beat from the left ventricle and measured in ml/beat. Stroke volume increases proportionally with exercise intensity.

Cardiac Output
Cardiac output is the amount of blood pumped by the heart in one minute, measured in L/min. It is the product of stroke volume and heart rate (SV * HR). If heart rate or stroke volume increases, cardiac output increases as well. Cardiac output increases as the intensity of exercise increases.

Blood Flow
During intense exercise, blood is redirected from organs – such as the kidneys, liver, stomach, and intestines – towards the skin, in order to promote heat loss.

Blood pressure
During exercise systolic pressure typically increases. However, diastolic pressure changes very little regardless of the intensity of exercise.

Risk Factors Favorably Modified by Physical Activity Habits

The National Center for Chronic Disease Prevention and Health Promotion reports that the use of physical activity in reducing rates of disease and death from chronic diseases has been well established. It's estimated that up to 580,000 annual deaths are related to poor diet and physical inactivity. Physical inactivity is also a major contributor to disabilities that result from chronic diseases such as diabetes, osteoporosis, obesity, and stroke.

Physically inactive people are almost twice as likely to develop coronary heart disease as people who engage in regular physical activity, according to The National Center for Chronic Disease Prevention and Health Promotion. In fact, the risk for heart disease is almost as prominent in individuals with physical inactivity as those individuals who smoke, have a high blood pressure, or have a high cholesterol level; and physical inactivity is more common than any of these other risk factors.

Obesity majorly contributes to various health problems including hypertension, dyslipidemia, Type II diabetes, coronary heart disease, stroke, gall bladder disease, osteoarthritis, sleep apnea, respiratory problems, and some cancers. Physical activity and proper eating habits are two of the most critical tools to fight obesity.

Individuals with risk factors for chronic disease such as hypertension or elevated cholesterol levels may be able to postpone or even prevent the onset of disease by integrating physical activity into their lifestyle. Individuals who have already developed a chronic disease can use physical fitness as a way to control the progression of disease.

Encouraging the integration of physical activity into an individual's lifestyle may be accomplished in numerous ways. Teaching them how to set goals, ways to build social support within their environment, how to reward themselves for achievements, and how to develop problem-solving skills are all ways to modify risk factors.

Adaptations to Exercise
Adaptions related to exercise testing and training are various. They include: improved neuromuscular functioning, such as increased strength and balance; improved cardiorespiratory function, such as

improvements in endurance; and an improved **functional capacity** (also known as maximum heart rate); just to name a few.

Additional Knowledge to Cover

Before we continue with our review, let's take some time to reiterate the meaning of some key terms which you will see – not only in the rest of this section – but also on the test, and continually throughout your career.

Lipoproteins

Lipoproteins are compounds made from a fat (lipid) and protein, and they transport cholesterol throughout the body via the bloodstream. There are four major lipoproteins produced by the body:

- **VLDLs**: Very Low-Density Lipoproteins. VLDLs travel through the bloodstream, losing some lipids while picking up cholesterol.

- **Chylomicrons**: Tiny lipoproteins classified as VLDLs.

- **LDLs**: Low Density-Lipoproteins. As VLDLs travel through the bloodstream, they lose some lipids, pick up cholesterol, and become LDLs. These distribute cholesterol to those cells in the body which require it.

- **HDLs**: High-Density Lipoproteins. Frequently referred to as good cholesterol, HDLs help remove bad cholesterol from the blood.

Although lipoproteins have a pivotal role in the body, they can also pose a health risk in certain situations. As VLDLs and LDLs move through the bloodstream and blood vessel walls, cholesterol can become stuck; and if enough cholesterol gets stuck, an artery may become clogged. This will eventually result in decreased blood flow, which can ultimately lead to a heart attack or stroke.

HDLs contain more protein than lipids and are therefore denser than LDLs. This density makes it tougher to penetrate the walls of blood vessels. As a result, HDLs aren't able to deposit cholesterol in vessels and instead transport it out of the body. This is why HDLs are considered *good* and why LDLs are often referred to as *bad*.

There are various factors which influence lipid and lipoprotein profiles. Some of these include:

1. **Heredity**: A family history of high cholesterol or heart disease increases the risk of developing these conditions.

2. **Diet**: Foods that are high in cholesterol, saturated fat, and trans fat increase cholesterol levels, which will likely be reflected in lipid and lipoprotein profiles.

3. **Body Weight**: Excess weight and obesity have been associated with high cholesterol levels.

4. **Physical Activity**: Exercise increases HDL levels, which lowers risks of heart disease.

5. **Age**: The risk of high cholesterol increases as individuals grow older.

The National Cholesterol Education Program, the American College of Cardiology, and the American Heart Association recommend the following diet and lifestyle changes to battle abnormal blood lipid profiles:

1. A diet low in total fat, saturated fat, and cholesterol, but high in fiber.

2. Weight management or weight loss if indicated.

3. Increased physical activity.

4. Smoking cessation.

5. Daily dose of low-dose aspirin.

High-Density Lipoprotein Cholesterol (HDL-C)
HDL cholesterol is frequently referred to as *good* cholesterol, because it offers protection against heart disease. HDL cholesterol helps remove *bad* cholesterol from the blood, which reduces build-up in the arteries.

An HDL number of less than forty for men and less than fifty for women is considered average. An HDL value of less than forty is considered a major risk factor for cardiovascular disease. An HDL value of sixty or more is optimal.

HDL Cholesterol Level	Value
Men and Women: 60 and Above.	**High**: Linked with lower risk of heart disease.
Men: Less than 40. Women: Less than 50.	**Low**: Linked with increased risk of heart disease.

Low-Density Lipoprotein Cholesterol (LD-L-C)
LDL is often referred to as *bad* cholesterol. It can build up on the walls of your arteries and over time result in the development of heart disease. Doctors often recommend that individuals with diabetes or other risk factors associated with heart disease strive for an LDL value of less than 100.

LDL Cholesterol Level	Value
< 100	Optimal
100 – 129	Very Good
130 – 159	Borderline High Risk
160 – 189	High Risk
≥ 190	Very High Risk

Total Cholesterol (TC)
The total cholesterol (TC) number is the number of milligrams of cholesterol in a deciliter of blood (mg/dL). This measurement includes levels of LDL cholesterol, HDL cholesterol, and other lipid elements.

Physicians recommend TC levels below 200. A TC number between 200 and 239 is considered mildly elevated. A TC number at or above 240 may require a complete fasting lipoprotein profile to more closely look at the condition.

Total Cholesterol	Value
< 200	Optimal
200 – 239	Slightly High
≥ 240	High

TC/HDL-C Ratio
Some physicians monitor an individual's TC/HDL-C ratio to determine how much of the total cholesterol value is composed of heart-healthy HDL in comparison to heart-unhealthy components of LDL and triglycerides. A low TC/HDL-C ratio is desired. The lower the ratio, the less risk an individual will likely have of suffering a heart attack or stroke.

Hyperlipidemia
This word is the medical term for high blood cholesterol. It commonly refers to high cholesterol and high triglyceride levels.

Student Tip: **H**DL Cholesterol = ***Healthy***. LDL Cholesterol = ***Lethal***.

Triglycerides
Food is converted to fatty acids and glycerol and stored within the body in the form of **triglycerides**. Hormones control the release of triglycerides from fat tissue. Elevated triglycerides can result from obesity, physical inactivity, cigarette smoking, excessive alcohol consumption, or a diet high in carbohydrates. People with high triglycerides frequently also have a high total cholesterol level. Individuals with the chronic diseases of heart disease or diabetes commonly exhibit high triglyceride levels.

Triglycerides Level	Value
< 150	Normal
150 – 199	Slightly High
200 – 499	High
≥ 500	Very High

The National Cholesterol Education Program (NCEP) was created in 1985 by The National Heart, Lung, and Blood Institute (NHLBI) to fight the illnesses and deaths linked with coronary heart disease (CHD). The recommendations of the NCEP are endorsed by over 40 leading health organizations including the American College of Cardiology, American Academy of Family Physicians, American Medical Association, American College of Preventive Medicine, and American Heart Association.

Recommendations of the NCEP include:

- All adults 20 years and over should have their serum cholesterol concentrations measured.
- HDL cholesterol levels should also be measured in addition to the serum cholesterol testing.
- This testing by a primary care physician will hopefully allow for the assessment of CHD risk of individuals and offer opportunities for interventions to reduce the risks at the time of detection.

Atherosclerosis

Atherosclerosis, broken down, means "hardening of the arteries," and occurs when cholesterol becomes stuck to the wall of the blood vessel, depositing and forming plaque in the arteries.

Early forms of atherosclerosis can be present as early as the ages of 20 and 30, though complications during these ages are rare. Lifestyle choices and risk factors such as smoking and obesity work to impair the function of arteries – even at these early ages.

In men after age 50, the rate of atherosclerosis development accelerates significantly. In women, accelerated risk occurs at age 60. After the age of 60, progressive atherosclerosis is prevalent. Arteries lose their flexibility and complications from atherosclerosis become a critical risk.

Exercise is one of the most significant ways to reduce the onset and progression of atherosclerosis, as it increases high-density lipoprotein (HDL), reduces blood pressure, reduces inflammation in the arteries, and helps maintain a healthy weight.

*Student tip: You will be asked on the exam about whether or not a client should proceed with a given exercise program based on test results which are given to you. Make sure you know the ACSM coronary risk factors and stratification information (information designed to increase safety of exercise training and efficacy of secondary prevention). Know how to use the risk factors as they apply to a real case study.

Test Your Knowledge: Pathophysiology and Risk Factors

1. True/False: Exercise lowers blood sugar levels in those with diabetes.

F 2. Exercise lowers blood pressure by keeping the walls of the arteries less flexible.

3. To estimate your maximum heart rate, subtract your age from what number?
   a) 125.
   b) 220.
   c) 200.

4. Coronary artery disease can lead to all of the following except:
   a) Heart attack.
   b) Emphysema.?
   c) Heart failure.
   d) Arrhythmias.

5. True/False: An adult over the age of 20 has several blood pressure readings below 116/80 mm Hg while at rest. He likely has hypertension.

6. True/False: Common symptoms of hyperglycemia include increased urination and thirst.

7. True/False: Pain, swelling, and redness of the joints are frequent symptoms of osteoarthritis.

8. True/False: The greatest exercise risk for individuals with diabetes is hypoglycemia.

9. True/False: Exercise-induced bronchospasm occurs when the airways in the lungs expand during exercise.

10. The National Cholesterol Education Program recommends that all adults __ years and over should have their serum cholesterol concentrations measured.

Test Your Knowledge: Pathophysiology and Risk Factors – Answers

1. **True**.

2. **False**. Exercise keeps the walls of the arteries more flexible.

3. **b)**.

4. **b)**.

5. **False**. The American Heart Association guidelines indicate that normal blood pressure readings for an adult over the age of 20 should be less than 120/80 mm Hg.

6. **True**.

7. **False**. These are symptoms of rheumatoid arthritis.

8. **True**.

9. **False**. This condition occurs when the lungs shrink during exercise.

10. **20**.

Final Thoughts

In the end, we know that you will be successful in earning your ACSM CHFS certification. Although the process can be challenging, if you continue with hard work and dedication, you will find that your efforts will pay off.

If you are struggling after reading this book and following our guidelines, we sincerely hope that you will take note of our advice and seek additional sources for help.

Start by asking friends about the resources that they are using. If you are still not reaching the score you want, consider getting the help of a tutor.

We wish you the best of luck and happy studying.

Most importantly, we admire your drive to enter into the health field – you are putting a lot of work into getting there. Your efforts are sure to pay off.

Sincerely,
The Trivium Test Prep Team

32248137R00136

Made in the USA
Lexington, KY
17 May 2014